NATURAL
BODY
NATURAL
MIND

NATURAL BODY NATURAL MIND

HEALTH, ECOLOGY
AND THE HUMAN SPIRIT

BILL TARA

Copyright © 2008 by Bill Tara.

Library of Congress Control Number:	2008902053
ISBN: Hardcover	978-1-4363-2736-7
Softcover	978-1-4363-2735-0

All rights reserved. No part of this book may be reproduced or transmitted in any form or by any means, electronic or mechanical, including photocopying, recording, or by any information storage and retrieval system, without permission in writing from the copyright owner.

This book was printed in the United States of America.

To order additional copies of this book, contact:
Xlibris Corporation
1-888-795-4274
www.Xlibris.com
Orders@Xlibris.com

Contents

Introduction 11

Health, Ecology, and Affinity

Chapter One: The Living Earth 17

Chapter Two: The Authentic Self 26

Chapter Three: Having or Being? 31

Chapter Four: The Question of Consciousness 40

Chapter Five: Health and Sickness 50

Chapter Six: Lessons of Wind and Water 60

Chapter Seven: Health and Habit 69

Natural Body / Natural Mind

Chapter Eight: Food and Culture 81

Chapter Nine: Food and Health 95

Chapter Ten: Body and Mind 108

Chapter Eleven: Five Archetypes 117

Chapter Twelve: Creating Balance 137

Chapter Thirteen: Strategies for Well-Being 155

Index 171

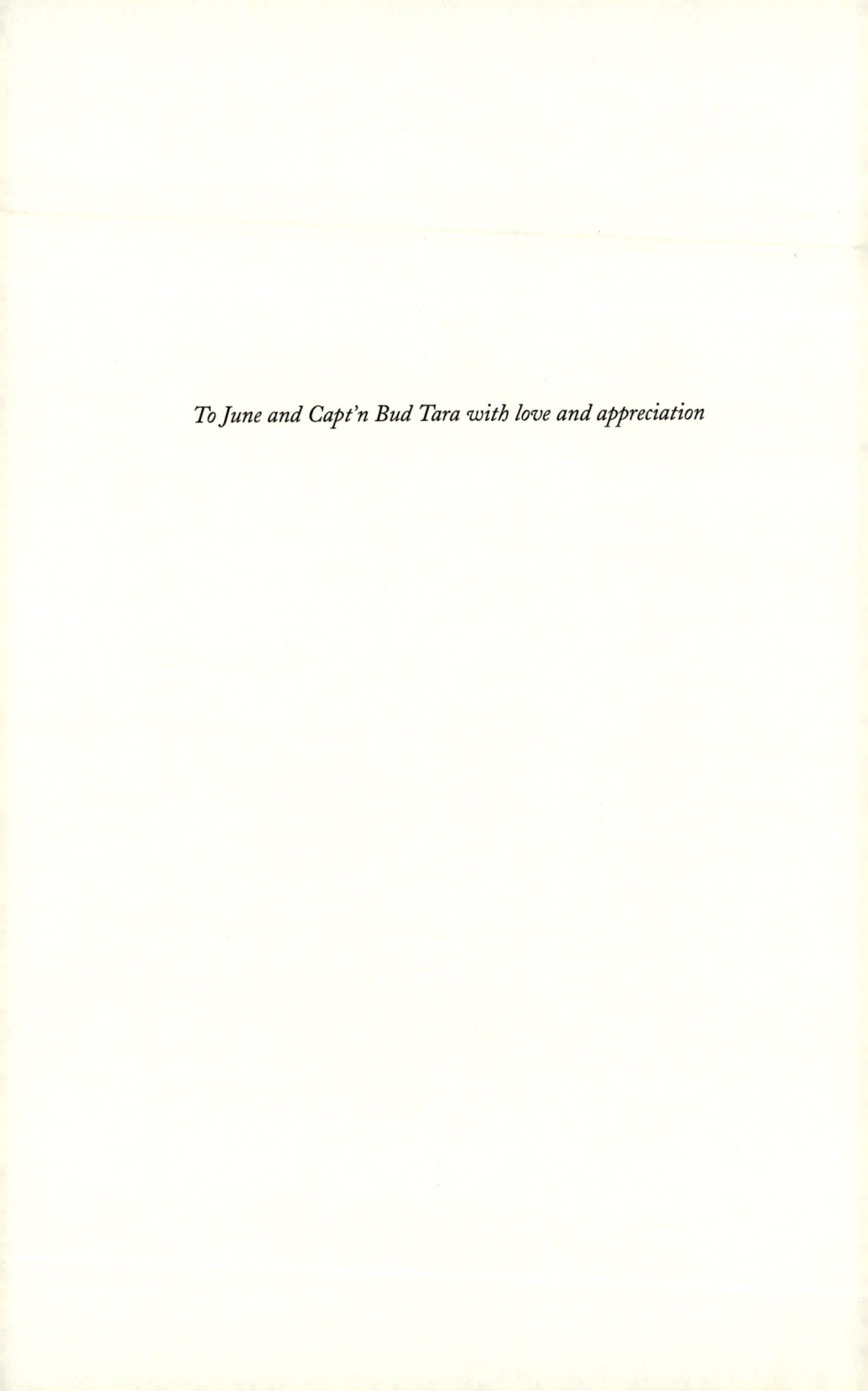

To June and Capt'n Bud Tara with love and appreciation

Acknowledgments

Over the years, the students who have attended my workshops and seminars in many parts of the world have inspired me the most. It is the curiosity, commitment, and sense of adventure that they bring into my life that keeps me on my toes.

I would like to thank Catherine Jansen for allowing me to use one of her beautiful works of art for the cover of this book. Please take a moment to visit her Web page for a full view of her astounding images: *www.catherinejansen.com*.

Finally to my wife, love, companion, and friend, Marlene Watson-Tara, for the humor, support, and good food she supplies daily.

Introduction

As a young boy growing up in Northern California, I was blessed with the opportunity to hike and camp in the woodlands of the Sierra Nevada and coastal ranges and to roam the rugged coastal cliffs and beaches. One of the highlights of every winter was when my father would take me to cliffs to watch the salmon returning to the river of their birth.

The rains would come, and the rivers would start to swell, and the salmon would gather off the coast. Standing on the cliffs, we could watch them swirl the water, silver in the reflected sun. They were coming back to renew the cycle of life. That they returned each year was miraculous and exciting. When the rains finally broke through the sandy mouth of the river, they would stir and leap into the silt brown waters to finish their journey. It never failed to make my heart race. It is a great sadness that my children and grandchildren will never see that sight.

The river has been altered from its former path. It has been widened and made shallow. Its banks have been dozed into levees to withstand an imagined flood. It is filled with grasses and algae—dank and unwholesome. The fish have been killed. Most of those coastal rivers are dead now. All the government studies in the world will not bring them back.

I do not know whether my daughters and sons will be able to hold their children's hands and watch the owl at dusk or the fox in the thicket. I do know that if they can't, their lives will be reduced in a very fundamental way. How we value nature says much about who we are. It speaks directly to the way we live our lives and the significance we place on our actions.

It has become all too common to say that the despoiling of our environment is the price of progress. If this is so, we need to ask what this supposed progress has brought us. If we are healthier, then why do we need ever-increasing numbers of hospitals and more drugs in order to function? If we are happier, why do more and more people complain of stress, and why are an escalating number of children prescribed with antidepressants?

Human history presents a sad portrait of our collective behavior. For every simple act of kindness, beneficial discovery, or creation of beauty, the scale is tipped dramatically by acts of brutality and stupidity on a massive scale. The qualities of violence, greed, and selfishness are dominant in the grand scale of human affairs and lie in sharp contrast to the guidance of the saints and sages we claim to admire the most. There is a deep disconnection between our stated humanity and our collective action.

Attempting to understand and explain this gap between our higher ideals and our most repellent actions has been the driving force behind religion, philosophy, and psychology. The troubling nature of our collective dementia has never before been this close to a critical breakdown. This collapse is not simply the result of new technologies of violence, escalating pollution, or increasingly sophisticated methods of political and economic suppression. The crisis we face is the suicidal destruction of the planet we inhabit. We are burning down the house and have no place to move.

The scope of this disastrous situation and the speed of its development create a special urgency to face the consequences of our actions and to alter the behavior that created them. We cannot solve the problems of unwise political, economic, and technological decisions with the same mind-set and through the same institutions that created them in the first place. A different way of thinking is required, thinking that may lead us to truths that are not only inconvenient but also exceedingly uncomfortable. The good news is that the challenge we face could provide us all with an astounding opportunity to transform human life on the planet in a beautiful way.

This book is about how our ideas, habits, and actions affect personal, social, and environmental health. I have tried to show the connection between these elements that are often separated by convention but not by fact. I have drawn on both ancient and modern sources since the roots of the problem are not new or simply a failure of modern technology but speak directly to our defining values. The foundation of the dilemma lies in our lack of a philosophy of life that serves to guide us toward healthy solutions. While modern medicine, science, and philosophy are good at reducing problems into discrete packets of data for analysis, it is the ancient ways of understanding that can provide better instructions of how to use this information wisely.

I make several assumptions that the reader should be aware of. The first of these assumptions is that our daily thoughts and actions have a profound effect on our health and well-being. We know that our diet, our environment, and our emotions are intimately linked to health. The second assumption takes us a step further. It is the notion that our state of health reflects our personal and cultural attitudes regarding human identity and our relationship with nature. The issues of personal, social, and environmental health are really only one issue. They are stages in the continuum of life process. When dysfunction is present in any stage of this continuum, the effects ripple out and infect the whole process.

Faced with the reality of increased sickness in individuals, nations, and the planet, we are forced to look clearly at the social institutions and cultural forces that resist a remedy. This sickness is not a conspiracy by hidden forces, but it is an act of protecting the status quo regardless of the results. I have used the issue of food in this book as an obvious example of how the habits of contemporary culture impact global health on all levels.

The growth, transportation, manufacture, and consumption of food together with the air we breathe and the water we drink is our most intimate biological connection to nature. When our relationship with air, water, and food are distorted, the effects are ruinous. The simple issues of supplying healthy food to the world is often made complex by the vested interests of the global food industry and the self-important posturing of food scientists. Beyond the weekly deluge of new diets, nutritional scares, and concern over weight gain lay larger issues that color every aspect of our lives. Hunger could be reduced, poverty eased, diseases among the wealthy and the poor could be reduced through changes in our attitudes regarding what we eat. All that is needed is the willingness to embrace change.

That willingness needs to be motivated by a positive desire to expand the scope of our vision of what life is and to bring our lives into alignment with that vision. The purpose of the changes that I recommend is to live a fuller life, a life that is healthy, vital, and filled with exciting self-discovery. It is for that reason that I have used many of the ideas that are common to the macrobiotic approach to health.

In presenting the ideas and ideals of this philosophy, I have focused on the implications of macrobiotic living. I have concentrated on the ideas that serve not only the individual but also society and the planet. Over the forty years of teaching the philosophy and practice of this unique version of Chinese medicine, I find that most of the conclusions stand the test of simple logic common sense.

The Japanese philosopher George Ohsawa introduced macrobiotics to Europe and America in the 1950s. Since Ohsawa's time, the changes in family life, food quality, the environment, and the pressures of daily life have transformed the world we live in at an astonishing speed. These changes need to be taken into account in the application of his ideas. Many of the toxic chemicals that are now in our food, air, and water were not even invented during Ohsawa's life. During his life, stress was not even considered or spoken of as a causal factor in disease. We did not work as many hours, travel as far to work, or spend as much time watching television. Fifty years ago, most families sat down to eat together and ate meals that had been made at home, which is no longer the case.

For the sake of simplicity, I have not made constant reference to the work of Ohsawa, Michio Kushi, Herman Aihara, or any of the other macrobiotic teachers and authors who have actively promoted the macrobiotic philosophy. I am deeply indebted to all of them, and I hope that those ideas I have borrowed and made my own reflect the spirit of their work if not always the detail.

William Wallace Tara
Tavira, Portugal
2007

Health, Ecology, and Affinity

Chapter One

The Living Earth

The Enchantments

Enchantments animate vast areas of our cultural landscape. Our mythology, our religion, and our folk wisdom are full of stories of enchantment. Men are turned into pigs, cities are turned to stone, and beautiful maidens are trapped in citadels of thorns. Someone always has to make a bargain with the devil, the evil witch, or the treacherous imp for the curse to be cast. The enchanted are always fooled and blocked from the promise of their true potential, dependent on the one act that breaks the spell, the act that sets them free.

We may think that kind of magic is a thing of the past, a fantasy now only mentioned in love songs or carnival acts. It might seem that the magic has been stripped of its veil by science and logic. But today's magicians worship different gods and weave different spells. The results are still the same. The illusionary gift is still splendid, gleaming and beyond all dreams, the result is a handful of dust and a frozen soul.

Today's sorcerers weave the promise of control over life itself. Now you can live in a castle, own the most majestic transportation, be handsome beyond belief, dine on the finest food, and extend your sex life for as long as you want. It is our belief in these miraculous promises that sustains the enchantment. The promise is a life of abundance, comfort, and pleasure never imaginable in human history—but like any enchantment, there is a price to pay. It is a price that is extracted slowly and surely from the fathers and mothers and paid for most dearly by the daughters and sons. The price of the modern enchantment is exactly that, the lives of our children.

The enchantment counts on the bewitched to put wisdom behind them and bury any thought of the true value of the trade. It depends on the avarice and shortsightedness of the enchanted. The modern enchantment is much the same as it was in the past with some minor changes. The magicians are now in suits; they are well pressed, confident, and secure. They speak of reasonable solutions to problems; they call for the formation of committees and think tanks. They speak in statistics and ridicule feelings and worship facts. They count on the bewitched to buy the vision that is offered without asking questions.

The modern tempter holds forth images of a future, protected and secure, where labor saving devices smooth out the problems of life, where computers educate the children, and where there is "more" of everything. It is a world of abundance without end and where experts take care of the problems and where personal irresponsibility will be balanced by benevolent social institutions.

The spell we labor under allows us to think that we can live in a way that produces disease and be fixed by a doctor, use up the resources of the planet, and have them replaced by science. The spell tells us that God is on our side when the governments that represent us protect the strong and repress the weak. We know that these promises are illusions, yet we continue as if they were true. The delusions and the actions that grow out of them produce a sickness of both the body and the soul that requires healing at the deepest level.

Health describes the dynamic balance between all aspects of our being. Many of the struggles we face in today's society seem divorced from our individual condition but are not. Our individual state of physical, mental, and spiritual well-being is reflected in everything we do. As part of the larger organism of society, we each play a role in its formation. Our state of health influences how we act in the world and to the kind of enchantments we are drawn to.

The Battle of the Wizards

It is natural that some of the most passionate debates in modern culture revolve around religion and science. It is here where a major battle for the human future is being waged. A long-standing and uneasy truce for the monopoly of the human mind seemed to exist between these potent forces, but the truce has been broken—the ceasefire has ended.

As social and environmental problems have grown, the humanistic intellectual tradition of secularism has come under increasing pressure from religious groups all over the world. Many in the scientific community, particularly the modern Darwinists, have joined in the conflict. It is a battle that has profound implications on how we understand our potential to develop and evolve individually and socially. Much of this struggle has to do with our collective visions of creation.

To the religious, the issue of evolution has always been a thorny one. The core belief that a god created the world in a particular way as described in religious scripture makes any scientific description heresy. Holy scriptures are accepted on faith and must be accepted as written or their whole fabric unravels. The stability of the faith and its ethical precepts require total acceptance. Any social evolution or development must be justified according to scripture as interpreted by the learned of the faith. Religions are systems of belief in a god and present a vision of how we need to behave in order to be bound to that god. They claim to tell us how we came to be and what we need to do. Here is a direct quote from Rev. Jerry Falwell, who until his recent death was one of the most powerful religious and political figures in America.

"The Bible is the inerrant... living word of God. It is absolutely infallible, without errors in all matters pertaining to faith and practice, as well as in areas such as geography, science, history, etc." Some people may think that this is just the ranting of an overly excited fanatic, but it is instructive to remember that American candidates for national political office vied with each other to get his blessing. The self-proclaimed ministers of God claim exclusive rights to the realm of spirit, and to exist, they must represent the final truth. Unfortunately this puts them in direct conflict with science.

Science also represents itself as the definer of truth. The truth of science is supposedly based on a rigorous collection of facts and the organization of those facts into a comprehensive system. Like religion, it claims the ability to tell us what we are, who we are, and where we came from. For many years, science has been the covert religion of the world. It is where popular faith has been most strongly invested. When a problem of health, environmental danger, or even business occurs, it is rare to call in a priest, mullah, or rabbi to pray for a solution. Nothing brings hope for redemption like a PhD. Science claims to deal with the real world, not the ethereal realms of spirit.

The problem is that the material world and the world of spirit come into increasing conflict. This fact is particularly true in the arena of social issues. How societies make decisions regarding abortion or genetic research or the definition of social norms call the conflict to the forefront. This is not simply an issue of difference between studies of risk assessment as opposed to prayer. The humanist tradition developed an ideal that human beings could create healthy and just societies through the application of ethical principles and study divorced of religious influence. The aim of this activity was the conscious evolution of humanity. For many, this concept of social evolution came to be an adjunct to the biological evolution described by Darwin. This humanist dream has taken on a new twist among many influential scientists.

Here is a quote from the naturalist E. O. Wilson, one of the world's leading Darwinists:

> **Genetic evolution is about to become conscious and volitional, and usher in a new epoch in the history of life ... The prospect of this "volitional evolution"—a species deciding what to do about its own heredity—will present the most profound intellectual and ethical choices humanity has ever faced ... humanity will be positioned godlike to take control of its own ultimate fate. It can, if it chooses,**

> alter not just the anatomy and intelligence of the species but also the emotions and creative drive that compose the very core of human nature.

What is being discussed here is that you and I decide that science can do the job if we just agree to let them forge ahead. The "godlike" ability being referred to is the capacity of science to manipulate genetic material. The gods will not be the general population but a select scientific priesthood who lay claim to the ability to make changes in something that is very poorly understood. This prospect is a little like asking the fox to guard the chickens.

The options seem somewhat limited. Either we agree that understanding our identity is only possible through the limited confines of specific religious belief or we hand the problem over to science for a solution. The other two wizardly covens, business and politics, are more malleable and will trim their sails to suit the winds of change. It is worth mentioning here that politics and business are so closely knit that it is difficult to separate them. This is very true in the arena of both health and the environment where government protection of business interests always trumps individual and planetary well-being.

Both science and religion have much to answer for including the fact that science has aspirations of being godlike, and religion seems intent on shrinking God down to an angry and vengeful old man. This does not mean that the pursuits of intellectual inquiry or spiritual development should be abandoned. What is important is that we reorient our thinking in a way that demands an improved ethic to the uses of science and a reinvigorated approach to religion that is focused on spiritual experience as opposed to dogma. This is good news since we are designed to accomplish this very task. All that needs to be done is to realign ourselves with the power of our own creation and rethink our relationship to the planet we live on.

Making God Small

One of the most fascinating periods of human history is the era between 900 and 200 BCE. During this short span of years, a diverse group of philosophers and mystics made their presence known in parts of Asia, the Near East, and Eastern Europe. They included Socrates, Buddha, Confucius, Jeremiah, and Lao Tzu; they all shared similar interests and came to similar conclusions regarding the human condition. They believed in the human capacity to live lives that were guided by the natural spiritual impulses of compassion and gratitude for the gift of life. It is not that they invented these concepts; most of them were present in more primitive cultures. Their gift was to shape them to the times they lived in.

It is instructive to look back at the vision of that time in history since the major religions of the modern world find their birth there. Confucianism, Taoism, Hinduism,

Buddhism, and the birth of the Rabbinic Judaism, Christianity, and Islam all find their roots there. What exists in our modern times are nothing more than narrow interpretations of these traditions, often glossed over with centuries of superstition and manipulation. The core spirit has been lost to the detriment of us all.

Karen Armstrong, a noted author on religion, has written a book on this period called *The Great Transformation*. I quote here from the introduction:

> **All the traditions that were developed during the Axial Age pushed forward the frontiers of human consciousness and discovered a transcendent dimension in the core of their being, but they did not necessarily regard this as supernatural, and most of them refused to discuss it . . . . The sages did not seek to impose their own view of this ultimate reality on other people . . . . If the Buddha or Confucius had been asked whether he believed in God, he would probably have winced slightly and explained—with great courtesy—that this was not an appropriate question . . . . What mattered was not what you believed but how you behaved . . . . The only way you could encounter what they called "God," "Nirvana," "Brahman" or the "Way" was to live a compassionate life.**

These attitudes certainly fly in the face of what we see as religion today. Most religious leaders are more than willing to talk about God in detail. The architecture of heaven, the robes of angels, and the number of times we incarnate are all seemingly known and eagerly explained. It would also seem that imposing religion on others is a primary function of many modern religions. The focus is obviously on believing, not on being. It is important that we look for the common ground between the intellectual search for truth and the spiritual one. A good place to start might be with the definition of God.

I once heard a Native American say that in his tribe there was no word for God; the closest expression they had was something like "Great Wow"! That sums it up pretty well. I'm sure the Taoists of ancient China would agree. The Taoists said, "The Tao that is expressed in words is not the eternal Tao." The message was clear: when someone starts to describe the architecture of heaven, run for the hills. The spirit of creation can be felt and can be seen through the product of its action, but not in its entirety. If the spirit of creation (or whatever label we prefer) pervades all things, it cannot be analyzed or described in detail. We seem to want the issues of the spirit to be "bite sized." We reject the feast and settle for a snack. We refuse to look around ourselves and see that we already live in paradise—it is up to us if we want to make it hell.

If we accept that nature seems to display repeated patterns of process, we have to ask how they came to be. Without some order in nature, there could be no science. All information would be a jumble of abstract happenings. The silly rejection of the concept of design in nature is almost as absurd as the idea that the world was made in one hundred and sixty-eight hours. It is only when we come to value our thoughts as well as our feelings, our intellect as well as our intuition that we can find a middle way that embraces all of our innate human capacities.

Even the Darwinists, when faced with the fact that not all human action can be explained through biological evolution, have been forced to speculate on the role of ideas, ideals, feelings, and cultural expressions such as art and music as driving forces in the unfolding of human potential. The fact that these phenomena exist beyond the realm of measurement of proof seems to not pose a problem. The idea of memes, invisible thought viruses, has caught the attention of some within the scientific community. The problem is that these memes are surely based on feelings. The most consistent feelings expressed in primitive as well as modern culture are that below the surface of the material world, there is a force that orders and creates all things.

What modern science has discovered through the application of technology and mathematics our ancestors discovered through personal experience. Life is much more an art than a science. It is an accepted scientific fact that the world we perceive is an illusion. All matter is comprised of energy vibrating at different speeds and forming an endless variety of compositions. Our normal perception scans the surface of this wonderful and ever-shifting display. Some of our ancestors dug deeper. Understanding the patterns and shifting tempos of the movement of energy held the secret of living well for them. They did not experience nature as a place of chaotic and arbitrary conflict but as a well-ordered pattern of relationships.

The ultimate source of this energy is of little interest to me. Like the Taoists, I feel that any attempt to describe something that lies beyond duality and contains all things within it is outside the realm of any concept I could imagine. Words like *god* or *infinite love* or *the power of creation* could all be translated into "too big to imagine." Fortunately we have the ability to see what happens when this primal energy divides itself into opposites. We know the unknowable by what it does. We may not see it, but we can feel it, and like a presence in a darkened room, we are aware that it is there. Since the unknowable permeates the totality of the material world, we can see the patterns of its movements and follow them like footprints in the sand.

The enchantment of both religion and science can limit our view rather than broaden it. Both lay claims to the truth as set by certain restrictions of logic, both can limit our capacity to be whole—to be healthy. When the world is defined as an accidental clump of chemical compounds, the larger potential of our lives is diminished. If we are here to simply worship God for a future reward, then we act out of fear. It is these deep streams of belief that are central to our relationship to nature and the ways in which we either honor or disdain it. Our capacity to alter the environment we live in is not unique. All living creatures do that. It is within humankind that this ability is most dramatically and often dangerously displayed.

Gaia

In the late 1960s, Professor James Lovelock published his Gaia hypothesis. His work focused attention on the fact that the planet Earth functioned as a single organism that maintains the perfect conditions for survival of both plant and animal life. Lovelock predicted many of the effects of global warming that are now accepted and put forward a way of seeing the world that was new to the scientific community. His ideas were ridiculed at the time but now are accepted as fact. His premise was not new. In fact, many primitive cultures embraced this notion. The difference being that their belief was based on experience, not theory.

The planet that we live within is just like each of us, an organism. It is not *like* an organism, it *is* an organism. We do not live *on* it—we live *in* it. We are a part of its structure, a group of its cells, and an organ in its body. It is important to know this and, even more important, to experience it. We are interacting with nature every moment. The flow of molecular energy in the water we drink, the food we eat, and the air we breathe represent a flow of energy that is continuous. The planetary environment courses through us—we are not the beginning or the end of this process.

The ancient Greeks named our planet-organism Gaia. They knew that she gives life to all things. The rivers and oceans, the hills and forests are all part of her body. Out of her, all life springs. She is Spirit made solid; she is a miracle of connections and rhythms, amazing creations, and wild force. Pictures of Gaia from space show a beautiful blue-and-green sphere floating in blackness. Those pictures presented to us the reality of our place in the vastness of the solar environment. We saw the beauty of our home, the oceans, the forests, and the spirals of cloud.

We can begin to see how the organism, Gaia, processes energy through distinct organ systems and transforms it for her own health, maintenance, and evolution. These processes, just like those in our own bodies, continue to move unattended, subtly working their wonder without intervention.

We are the earth—the earth is us. It is the secret of the stone, the stream, the seas of grass that they move within us. Our identity is not so small that we can write it on a single page. We do not cease to exist at the surface of our skin. We are permeable. When we are enveloped by nature, awash in the sounds of bird and breeze, when we breathe the smell of dry leaves or fresh grass, we are home and know it.

The crust of the earth with its undulating system of mountains, valleys, and plains provides Gaia with her skeletal system. It is a flexible system just like ours. It can adapt to the movement of the planet as it races through the solar system. Gaia doesn't just sit in space, she moves, she dances. She contracts and expands, adapting to the force of her journey around the sun and her larger sojourn through the galaxy. The earth's crust serves the same function as the bones in your spine or rib cage. It provides structure and support for movement.

I have sat high in the Rocky Mountains and looked at the rise and fall of the range in the distance. From the high places, you can see how these peaks moved up through the crust of the earth. In the mind's eye, you can feel the upward thrust and the peeling away of the surface—such force, such power. Continents are born, mountains are plunged in the sea, new lands rise up, and the old are buried. Bone is the stone the body makes. Dust of stones, pulled up by the roots of plants, eaten by us, fixed in us as nail and bone. We hold the stones of the earth within us.

In her infancy, comets and asteroids partly made of frozen vapors bombarded Gaia. This was the seed food, the source of the primitive atmosphere and seas. Together with radiation from the sun and carbon dioxide released from beneath the surface of the planet, an atmosphere was born, and clouds were formed.

No one really knows how the ancient seas arose from the atmosphere. They may have been produced from the distillation of original gases and water or from the melting of ice. The leaching of minerals from the rocky base, the surging volcanic activity, and the new seeding of comets and asteroids enriched these ancient seas. The blood of the planet was this nutrient-rich sea, out of which all life was born.

The seas were the beginning of a circulatory system that moves fluids through the biosphere. Evolving from these most ancient seas, the circulatory system is now comprised of a complex network of lakes and rivers interconnected with each other both above—and below ground. These are the veins, arteries, and capillaries of the planet, which allow fluids to circulate through the Gaian biosphere, cleaning it and reconstituting it in the process. The waters of Gaia are the foundation of both plant and animal life. They comprise the major substance of our body and all living things.

The very same rivers and seas flow within us. The tidal rush of blood bathes the cells, washes against the walls of our being. These tides fill the spiral conch of the ear, they form the magic gel of the eye, and we see and hear through these waters. Pulled by the moon, drawn by the sun, the pulse of this tide moves our heart. The seas of Gaia move within us all.

Forests and grasslands provide Gaia with a respiratory system. They cycle the gases of the planet and purify them in the process. Without the great forests and grassy plains, we would have no air to breathe; without the process of photosynthesis, there would be no food chain. Your lungs and the leaves of plants are a mirror image of each other. The plant takes in the respiratory waste material of the animal, carbon dioxide, and in exchange releases oxygen for the animal kingdom to breathe. Plant life takes in the environment directly—combining minerals, water, and radiation from the sun to form the nutrients that all animal and insect life need to thrive.

Plants first ventured onto the stone from the seas. They changed the chemistry of the atmosphere and grew on the rocky shores and slowly, slowly crept to cover all the spaces exposed. Without the brotherhood of plants, we die. There is no creature, scaled, feathered, or covered with fur that does not owe its daily food to the miracle of the breathing leaf.

Soil is the digestive system of the planet. The primitive soil was created from the decomposition of dying plants and animals. As plant life claimed the dark and silent stone, it lay down its substance to form the medium for new life. The top six inches of soil creates one of the most fundamental systems for all life on the planet. Without it, there would be no life on the land. Within the soil live the millions of microorganisms that digest plant and animal matter and create the potential for plant growth and the beginning of the food chain. These tiny creatures aerate the soil and fix plant nutrients; they recycle matter and bring it back to the service of life.

From microorganism to Homo sapiens, the more complex life-forms evolved. Those that swim and fly, those that roam the jungles or live deep within the soil represent a movement toward something more abstract, something with a beautiful and dangerous gift. We are different yet share our origin; we are as distinct as the heart is from the lung yet part of one body.

The process of evolution can be perceived as the development of increased complexity of structure and level of organization, which proceeds from the basic energetic interactions of subatomic particles into the organization of the basic elements, the vegetable kingdom, and finally the cellular organization of the animal kingdom. This increased complexity reached its current pinnacle in the human structure and specifically the evolutionary developments of the brain. This is not to say that humankind is better or more important than all the rest of life on the planet, a notion sometimes wrongly taken. What it does indicate is a particular kind of difference, a particular quality of being that holds a stunning potential if used well.

Chapter Two

The Authentic Self

The Gift of Life

The unknowable power of creation gives the gift of life. It is only when we honor this gift that we come into our true potential, our true self. Even those in pain reach out to this feeling of being one with the creative force of life. Access to that gift is always present and available. The fourteenth-century mystic Meister Eckhart had this to say about it:

> **You need not seek him here or there, he is no further off than at the door of your heart: there he stands lingering, awaiting whoever is ready to open and let him in. He longs for you a thousand fold more urgently than you for him.**

Here is the interesting part: "he (The Unknowable) longs for thee a thousand fold more urgently than thou for him." If Eckhart is right, we have to assume that the unknowable has some need that we accept and become one with it. We do not have to think of this in terms of human desire but rather that there is an urge toward creation and completion. The physicist Niels Bohr said,

> **If I was a molecule and I wanted to know what I was I would have to create a human being.**

Could it be that Gaia has an urge to do something like that? Is it possible that through human consciousness the whole earth becomes self-aware? It is a question worth asking.

The Authentic Self

When we feel the power of our connection with the source of our being, we are more alive and more present to the moment. We can think of this as a state of emotional affinity. It is a state where we are attracted to and share an identity with the person, place, or thing that we perceive. It is not an intellectual process, it is felt. One of the characteristics of our modern life is a "hardening of boundaries" that creates a barrier to the affinity we long for. This is a form of isolation that is endemic to modern culture, the futurist Faith Popcorn labeled it "cocooning." A softening of boundaries works in the opposite direction.

The softening of boundaries is a state of being where the usual limits of our sense of self dissolve, and for a moment, we don't know where we end and the rest of the world begins. This state of being is not madness, but it is not "normal." It is an extraordinary experience, an event that broadens the consciousness. It serves to expand and deepen our appreciation of life, and relationship to the world we live in. It is our experience of being one with our creation. It is not necessary to imagine the extreme state of ecstasy as the ultimate goal. Excitement, joy, happiness, peacefulness, and simply being one with the moment all take us out of the perplexing anxieties that characterize modern life and transport us into a different way of seeing and feeling.

Softening our boundaries can occur in a heartbeat with no warning. A loved one, a flight of birds, or a beautiful song can trigger it. When we experience this oneness, we know who we are in a unique way. The experience, even if a brief one, strips away our identity as a name, an occupation, or an estimate of net worth. It takes us into the heart of an astonishing paradox. We are humbled by our smallness, and yet our identity is enlarged. We may rightfully feel blessed when this happens, and it has happened to everyone. It is the single experience that has most occupied human religion and philosophy since before written history and is the driving force behind most great art. It is the search for the sacred. It may have little to do with organized religion and yet is the bedrock of a spiritual life.

While we have all experienced the softening of boundaries that characterize the sacred qualities of life, we often don't know what to do with the event. We don't know how to express it or, more importantly, how to consciously call it back. This is particularly true when we realize that these experiences most often occur in childhood before we have been told how the world is "supposed to be." In many primitive cultures, this experience was revered and nurtured. It may have even qualified a person for a special position in the tribe or family. In some societies, this experience has been demonized, thought to be a dangerous sign of insanity, an aberration of the childish imagination, or the work of the devil.

This is ironic since the men and women who are most admired in the world for their spiritual insight—the avatars, saints, wise women, prophets, and sages—spent their whole lives talking about this experience. They sought out ways to consciously access this state of being and to cultivate it. They created a vocabulary to understand its working and sets of skills to call it forth. These states of being were and are valued because it is an experience of the self without the conceptual and cultural trappings that hold us in the confines of daily life. It is the experience of our authentic self.

The archives of spiritual traditions throughout the world and the rich wisdom of tribal stories are filled with instructions defining the mind-set and physical techniques that can be called into service to this end. These practices covered the whole territory of human experience from how to cope with death to how to give birth, from systems of physical control and martial arts to creating a meaningful sex life. This wisdom is often embedded in legend, myth, or songs that serve as guideposts for the journey into an expanded and deepened consciousness. From the mundane to the sublime, this wisdom was aimed at opening the doors to the experience of oneness. The poet, the artist, or the mystic may tumble gracefully into this state of perception naturally, but to benefit fully, some degree of self-mastery is essential.

When we live in harmony with nature, we move toward the authentic self. Our sensitivity is heightened and our intuition sharpened. The scientist or physicist may speak about electrons and molecules, but the authentic self feels that the movement of the life force requires a different set of concepts that engage our total being and not just the activation of the mind. The only problem with this is that when we move into our own authenticity, we can find ourselves out of synch with much of the culture that surrounds us.

The Natural Mind

Many think that the experience of the authentic self is a mysterious process for only the enlightened few. The great spiritual thinkers disagree. The great spiritual teachings show that having the experience of "oneness" is available to everyone. It is our birthright to be whole in body and spirit. The fact that we do not experience our personal softening of boundaries is due to the fact that we are held back by the way we live our lives. The treasure is hidden in full sight. It is in the grain of sand, the mustard seed, in the sound of one hand clapping. We are built for it.

The search for our innate desire to experience our oneness with nature is not only the province of myth and folk story. It is found in most religious texts, in the writing of poets, and the songs of minstrels; it flows through Henry David Thoreau and Walt Whitman and animates the early writers on ecology such as Rachel Carson. It may start with an ecstatic moment or a flash of insight, but it always moves to absorb the whole being. That search for oneness opens our eyes to the ways in which our human attitudes toward nature are deadened by a culture increasingly cut off from its roots. It unerringly leads to a vision of human ecology that can be found in many emergent movements that address a renewal of our bond with nature.

The vegan and vegetarian movements reflect our insensitivity toward animals; the organic farming movement reflects our lack of care for the soil. The surge of interest in protection of ancient growth forests or endangered species all speak in an urge to reunite our culture with the source of our being. They move in direct opposition to the view that the environment is something only there for our exclusive use. When we look at nature as simply a resource to feed our own appetites and to fuel our economies with no other inherent value, we align ourselves with the destruction of the planet. It is only when we see ourselves as totally dependent on nature as the source of our being that we can make the kind of personal and social actions that lead to a healthy outcome.

Our present culture and the enchantments that are its bedrock cannot supply the spiritual and physical nurture we so desperately need for our own health and development. By ignoring the visceral and spiritual requirement of natural harmony for a healthy life and a healthy planet, we become strangers in our own land. We are lost without a map to guide us or a compass to point the way. It is precisely this estrangement, this physical and spiritual emptiness that creates the hunger for the consumer goods, the junk foods, and the mindless entertainment and celebrity dramas of modern living. When this hunger is fed with ideas and objects that do not nourish the body, mind, or spirit, our search for satisfaction becomes more ravenous and desperate. We become addicted to those very things that pervert our true potential with the mistaken thought that more of the same will fill that spiritual void.

In Praise of Eccentricity

I have had the distinct pleasure to meet some powerful people in my life; most of them were just a little crazy. Their successes were firmly based on not doing what was normal, accepted, or expected. Their willingness to go against the grain of social norms was the key to their success. They all had the faith in their own authentic self to resist the oppressive effects that can be promoted by family or society or religion. For every one of these men and women, there are hundreds who do not find the inner strength to empower themselves. Rather than stimulating original thought, our social institutions are created to deflect the potential impact of the renegade especially when the idea challenges a favorite enchantment. We settle too easily into accepting the unacceptable.

Are we being encouraged to lead healthy and creative lives, or are we spurred onward to sickness and apathy? Are we taught that the only value of nature is as a source of base matter to fuel our immediate pleasure or to respect the diversity and beauty of life for its own sake? Are we cautioned to live simply or to live outside our means? Questions of this kind are essential because we often live within enchantments that are so pervasive that we can only see them by moving ourselves outside the fray. Society is always a leveler—conformity to the norm is expected and most often required. This fear of diversions to cultural alignment can be stifling to the evolution of group consciousness and usually serves only the vested interests of the powers that be.

If it is normal to be unhappy with your job, suffer from poor health, or be endlessly in debt, what is that attraction of normalcy? It is certainly more desirable to be abnormal in that case. The eccentric path invariably leads away from the central concepts and actions that define any culture. That path always defines a new center and puts forward a vision much different from the existing model. It also always provokes fear and even anger with those who cling to the old. The fear of change is an anchor that keeps us fixed directly in the path of the oncoming storms while we try desperately to bail out the water with very small buckets.

Mediocrity is the hallmark of this century. Mediocrity rules our culture from politics and religion through the arts. Big ideas have been traded in for small adjustments. Consider the absurdity of government environmental policies that encourage large polluting companies to trade toxic waste coupons with less polluting ones rather than demanding that all offenders conform to safe standards. Consider health care debates that never mention preventing diseases that are known to be preventable but focus on who will pay for the invasive treatment of those diseases when they occur. The only reason that these bland solutions to difficult problems are accepted is the fear that the real solution will mean mammoth change, not simply a little tweak.

I heard a Zen monk say that the moment of his satori was like a tadpole transforming into a frog. He said that this was why the enlightened soul had such difficulty expressing his or her experience. The tadpole lived only in the world of water, poking its nose up for air on occasion. The frog now lived in the world of air, a world where things were different.

While the frog knew the world of water and could live in it, he also knew the world of air, a world that could only be communicated to those who had shared the experience. There was no feeling of superiority in the monk's statement, but the constant twinkle in his eye and the purity of his humor said it all he was living mostly in the air. We have all experienced our tadpole period. It seems that we are a little scared of becoming a frog. We shouldn't be afraid—we might get kissed by a princess (or a prince as the case may be).

Chapter Three

Having or Being?

The Pursuit of Happiness

I have borrowed the name of this chapter from the title of an excellent book by Erich Fromm. During his life, Fromm was one of the most highly respected thinkers on philosophical and social issues. His book *To Have or To Be?* was published four years before his death in 1980. He reflected the view of many enlightened men and women of his generation that the direction of society was aimed not only at ecological disaster but also at the deadening of human experience. It was a book about the health of the mind and spirit.

What Fromm and others observed was that in the decades after World War II, human society in the West seemed to hasten all the worst aspects of its economic systems. The goal for the individual became the acquisition of property and money; these were seen as the attributes of success and value. None of this was new of course. The difference was that rather than being concentrated in the extremely rich, this affluence was now available to the rapidly growing middle class. The race was on. Societies in the West, primarily America, created a culture entirely focused on consumption. This consumption was not the acquisition of goods that were a lasting legacy; these were goods that were designed to be disposable. The fact that they were disposable was essential to feed the growth of the economy and produce the illusion of unlimited prosperity. The true price of this prosperity is only now surfacing in spite of the best efforts of government and business to delay the payment.

Dramatic rises in the cost of food and fuel, increased poverty among the already poor, and a continuing degradation of the natural environment will be problems that the next generation will inherit. The cost is already being paid by the continued rise in the costs of food and basic services all over the world as well as the disappearance of nature. All of this has taken place against the background of what has been described as a "growing economy."

Our concern with the abstraction we call "the economy" is the consistent reason put forth for inaction for environmental and health concerns. The assumption is that the growing economy will produce happiness. We have to believe that simple premise or the whole enterprise would be seen as foolish. The difficulty is that the relationship between affluence and happiness is proven wrong time and again.

This does not mean that deprivation and happiness go hand in hand. To the contrary, having the basics of a healthy life such as healthy food, shelter, clean water, and security are all essentials and describe the primary human needs. Every person on the planet should be assured of these. None of these cost much money compared to the cost of maintaining a system that denies them.

To believe in these ideals is not to be a socialist or a communist or a utopian. I feel compelled to say this since any critique of the current economic system seems to call up these tired old accusations to disarm or discredit. If we are to create a healthy world that provides at least the minimum requirements for well-being to the citizens of the planet, we will have to call forth the courage to question the causes of the problems and the will to take action.

The furrowed brows of public leaders as they tiptoe around this issue is a pathetic sight. When any critique of consumerism is broached in America, it is seen as an attack on the fundamental principles of the nation. When linked with environmental issues, it is easily seen as being the work of hippy communards, tree-hugging "environmental wackos," or Luddites. The denial of any relationship between the so-called free market and the consumerism it feeds are even perceived by some as unpatriotic.

The enchantment of endless bounty is one that has formed much of the philosophy of the market economy and now shows itself in the guise of spiritual teaching as well. We live in and on a planet that rivals any imaginable paradise, and yet we are encouraged in the belief that having a motorboat or a cell phone will improve it. The enchantment of endless bounty is a gross misinterpretation of the gift we have been given. Native people throughout the world have long known that the earth is here to be cared for and that when we ignore that simple fact, we suffer. This enchantment can only exist if we avoid exposure or deep reflection on its results. The paradox is that the consumption that we have been led to believe will produce happiness may well be the primary cause of our misery.

Psychologist Oliver James, author of *Britain on the Couch*, has done studies indicating that affluence has no impact on whether or not you are likely to be happy. His research also showed that "a 25 year old today is 5-10 more times likely to suffer from depression compared to a 25yr old in the 1950's." The wider implications of this, argues James, is that "the dominant values of Western Society are almost literally programming us to be unhappy."

In 2003, a World Value Survey of people in sixty-five nations was published in the British magazine *New Scientist*. The survey found that the world's happiest countries with the most satisfied people are Puerto Rico and Mexico, and those with the most optimistic people are Nigeria and Mexico; a later study put the residents of the island of Tobago on the list.

The results of surveys of this kind run counter to conventional wisdom. The notion presented by media hype and social conditioning equates prosperity with happiness. If that is true, how can people in these poorer nations be more content than prosperous Americans who scored an unimpressive sixteenth on the list? One thing is sure; the answer doesn't lie in the gross domestic product per capita. Estimates in 2003 showed the US with a GDP per person of $37,800. How does this compare with the world's happiest nations? GDP per person in Puerto Rico is $16,800; in Mexico, it is $9,000; in Nigeria, it is a pitiful $800.

Several of these countries suffer from poverty, corrupt government, and high rates of violence. There is no reason that we should wish those things on anyone, and yet they felt they were happy. A case could be made that their expectations were lower than other countries; it could be that they lied about their true feelings. There could be many reasons why the results of the survey could be wrong. This and other studies on happiness lie in sharp contrast to what we expect to be true except that there is compelling evidence that they are accurate. That evidence is found in the increasing incidence of depression and mental stress found among the affluent.

Depression is usually described as an illness that influences the body, thinking, and mood. It affects the way that people think about themselves and the world around them and has a profound influence on sleep patterns, sex, and eating. Feelings of hopelessness, worthlessness, fatigue, and restlessness are common. In the extreme, there is difficulty in decision making and thoughts of suicide. Over the past fifty years, the incidence of this disease has risen dramatically in the affluent countries of the world.

The causes of this problem have been put down to a loss of religious belief, exposure to toxic substances, financial stress, striving to meet unattainable personal or professional goals, and any number of the commonly experienced problems of modern living. While there is no accepted solitary cause for depression, there is one thing that is known without a doubt—it is affecting the young at a much higher rate than in previous times.

According to the Joseph Rowntree Foundation, the number of young people battling depression has doubled in the past twelve years. Similar studies in America by the National Institute of Mental Health estimated that over 10 percent of the population suffered from clinical depression. Children born after 1955 will suffer a major depression—not just sadness, but also a paralyzing sense of hopelessness—at some point in their lives at twice the rate of their grandparents' generation. These troubling facts could lead us to question the kind of culture we are creating because it seems to be driving us away from happiness rather than toward it.

In *To Have or To Be?* Fromm addressed the urgency of the issue over thirty years ago in the following way:

> **The need for profound human change emerges not only as an ethical or religious demand, not only as a psychological demand arising from the pathogenic nature of our present social character, but also as a condition for the sheer survival of the human race. For the first time in history the *physical survival of the human race depends on a radical change of the human heart.* However a change of the human heart is possible only to the extent that drastic economic and social changes occur that give the human heart the chance to change and the courage and the vision to achieve it.**

In describing the character of modern society, he uses the term *pathogenic*. We have created a culture that causes disease by its very existence. No matter what steps are taken to patch up the symptoms, the sickness is still there. We keep patching one problem, only to have it appear somewhere else. A frustrating dilemma unless your livelihood is patching things up as opposed to fixing things.

The wounds will not heal unless the underlying causes are clearly addressed. Fromm identified the crucial question as to whether we wanted our life to be about "being" or "having." The very idea that we might not be able to do both sends a shiver through the cultural cortex. Of course the choice is not quite that stark. We can still have plenty, but we certainly need to redefine what we want and very surely what we need.

We are faced with the dilemma of consuming less or consuming differently. It is a silly argument—we need to do both. So far it has not been demonstrated that the move to "green products" has curbed the desire to spend overall, it has simply created a new demographic for marketers to cater to. Increased purchase of designer shopping bags to replace the plastic ones is more of a culture statement than a wise use of resources. We need products with less environmental impact and with increased energy efficiency, but we are also required to use less of everything. Our crisis of personal and environmental health is not simply another marketing opportunity.

American psychologist Tim Kassar has analyzed all the studies done on the relationship between wealth and happiness and come to a startling conclusion: material gain does not ensure happiness. His studies indicate that

> **people who are primarily motivated by "materialism," (which in this case means the pursuit of power, status, wealth and possessions) are much more likely to be unhappy in almost every respect, including being less healthy than those who remain resolutely un-materialistic.**

The consumerism that dominates the culture of the industrialized world is firmly focused on distracting attention away from unhappiness. The pervasive disease of modern culture is not cancer; it is anxiety. It is fear of the unknown.

What would we do if we had to live in a smaller house? What would happen if we couldn't drive to work? What would happen if we couldn't get organic sun-dried tomatoes from that quaint village in Sicily? What would happen if an unknown terrorist group mysteriously destroyed all television signals?

When fear—real or imagined—dominates our lives, happiness cannot and will not appear. Fear is the major tool of advertisers and governments alike. You only need that expensive deodorant if you think you would stink without it. We only support policies that destroy the environment for the next generation if we are told that economic disaster will result if those policies change. It is the fear of change that allows us to accept the false promises of happiness on offer. The more we feed the beast, the more powerful it becomes.

The average person living in Western society is assaulted by thousands of advertisements each day. With millions of dollars of sophisticated market research at their command, advertisers can take advantage of consumer psychology to attract attention, penetrate resistance, and effect consumption with astounding success. Casting an enchantment doesn't come cheap. They have decoded the hidden needs of the human mind and addressed a fundamental flaw in the modern psyche—insecurity.

It is exactly our lack of self-confidence that feeds the machine of overconsumption. We want more of everything because we don't know if we will pass the test of close scrutiny. If the newest car or electronic toy gives us bragging rights or the newest style clothes give us the mark of cultural savoir faire, it might disguise the deep anxiety that, if stripped bare of our material trappings, we are just "not good enough." It is the emptiness of our lives that demands being filled with junk. Without an insecure population, the market is forced to provide only those goods and services that have real life-enhancing value.

When our social value is defined by the products we buy, the car we drive, and the amount of money we make, we find ourselves in a cycle of consumption to keep up at all cost. This is exactly the purpose of the marketplace—once we have bought into the market ideal, there is continual anxiety to maintain our place with "the next best thing." It is the Catch-22 of the market economy since as soon as you have the newest model, it needs to be replaced by a newer, more improved version. This model depends on an uneducated consumer; more accurately, one educated by advertising alone, a lack of ethical goals in production aside from bottom-line profit and the assumption of endless raw materials for production. It depends on individuals to accept the enchantment of a culture built on hollow and degrading promises or one built around a true concern for the long-term well-being of the citizenry.

What about Well-Being?

Any discussion of well-being must include a definition of the *being* part. My dictionary contains several options for *being*; the first of these is mere existence—the one I was looking for lies farther down the list. This definition says that *being* is "a state or condition of fully realized potentialities; the end point of the process of becoming." Ah, this is the issue at hand. *Being* means realizing our potential. When we speak of the development of humanity, have we reached the end point, or are we still in the process of becoming?

It seems that the image put forward by many is that we have arrived at the zenith of our evolution and chaos rules. Is it any wonder that we look for someone to come in and organize things, someone to clean house, and someone to make sense of it all? The ability of individuals to make any difference given the magnitude of the problem is negated. This negation of personal action does nothing but serve the purposes of institutions that are all too willing to accept the power to act on our behalf. If we look at the guiding principles of an earth-friendly economy, we can vision new and exciting ways to move beyond these apparent constraints. Creating a new vision of human health is an important part of this process.

I once attended a macrobiotic conference on cancer that featured about fifteen people who had been diagnosed with fatal cancer and were now in remission from the disease. Some of them had been declared cured by their doctors against all odds. The single comment that every one of them made at one point in their story was that being ill made them reflect on the true value of their life. Having cured themselves by changes in their lifestyle, they now saw their disease as the best thing that had happened to them. They had what Fromm referred to as "a radical change of heart." I have observed that when people are ill and heal themselves that the sense of empowerment is transformative.

There are those who believe that the same will be true with the environmental problems we are facing. They say wait till the ocean levels rise and the crops fail and the oil runs out, then people will act. Even Professor Lovelock seems to have given up hope for Gaia's future. In an interview with the *Guardian* newspaper, he dismissed most environmental work as a fantasy. I suppose after ringing the warning bell for over forty years, he has the right to be a little bitter, but one statement he makes is worth noting. He stated that the only kind of commitment that could change the tide was the kind that animated Europe in the years following World War II, when the situation was so bad that fear and desperation drove societies to rebuild in the wake of destruction. We need to hope that the same scale of collapse in the affluent countries of the world is not the essential spur to a change in direction.

Economy and *ecology* both spring from the same linguistic roots meaning the house or home. Ecology refers to "knowing" the home (how it works); economy has to do with managing the home. Economy is the task of wisely using the resources at hand. It might seem that our present predicament concerning the environment and the economy is that we have been lead into a false economy. Our present economy does not entail the wise use of our resources—in fact, it is driven and depends on the unwise use of them. Politicians of every stripe line up with regularity behind the idea that increasing the ability of the population's ability to spend more can solve all problems in Western society. The obvious problem here is that consumerism does not equate with happiness or fulfillment. Unbridled consumption is exactly the same as junk food—empty of nutritional value, designed to create a fleeting satisfaction, and promoting increased hunger.

Bread and Circuses

When the citizens of Rome had experienced just about enough poverty and squalor and were ready to riot the ruling classes had quick solution—free bread and a new circus at the coliseum. If the unruly masses had some food in their stomach and an afternoon of excitement and slaughter, the pressure would slack off, and the anger would be put to the side for a while. Slaves would be made to fight each other to the death, and exotic animals would be killed for pleasure. We are right to condemn that practice—it is barbaric. The problem is that it worked like magic.

We all love magic tricks. We love to see that card disappear from the hand or that pigeon fly out of a hat. The fact that we know that it's a trick doesn't spoil the joy of it. It all has to do with distracting attention and the skillful movement of the fingers. What should our response be if the same distractions were used to pull our attention away from the fact that we were about to get run over by a bus?

I invite you to watch "reality" TV or the sad profusion of daytime shows where people are set up for ridicule and humiliation for the sake of entertainment. What is this for if not to deflect attention from a desolate life? Bread and circuses have been replaced by fast food, celebrity culture, and television. To escape the stresses of work and the uncertainty of life in debt, the mind-dulling electronic media hum of corporate sponsorship presents the new Roman circus. The escape is not a cure for the malaise but a sedative—a reassuring reminder that everything is fine. The distractions keep us away from our true self and the experience of our true potential.

The times when we all feel most alive, most engaged with the moment are those that Mihaly Csikszentmihalyi, the former head of the department of psychology at the University of Chicago, has identified as being in "flow." This state can appear in any arena of life. It is when our involvement in the moment and the actions we are taking seemingly erase time and all other considerations. Here is how he describes it:

> **Happiness is not something that happens. It is not the result of good fortune or random chance. It is not something that money can**

> buy or power command. It does not depend on outside events, but, rather, on how we interpret them. Happiness, in fact, is a condition that must be prepared for, cultivated, and defended privately by each person. People who learn to control inner experience will be able to determine the quality of their lives, which is as close as any of us can come to being happy.

This state of being is most often experienced when we have goals that are exciting to us and can engage the attainment of those goals with total passion and commitment. It is within the creative tension between where we are and where we want to be that the potential exists for our most profound experience. The true colors of the human experience shine when we are engaged in the act of creation. This means that we must have belief in our own ability to move beyond the mundane and to create something with real value in our lives. It is essential that we recognize our potential as agents of positive change.

Ideas that guide us beyond the learned limits of our biology and our most basic emotional responses are essential. Our biology, sensitivity, and emotions are fundamental foundations to our state of being, but they are not the only engines that drive us forward. It is easy to look at human history and come to the sad conclusion that much of human behavior is driven by fear, greed, and aggression; but these are not ideas—they are emotions. Even when they are justified or ennobled by scientific or political theory, they still belong to a lower state of being. It would be absurd to think that a lasting, harmonious, or principled society could be built on that shaky footing. These archaic compulsions certainly exist, but they are not sufficient for realizing our full potential or for explaining the best of human endeavors. It is important that we establish firm bridges between the wisdom of the past and the promise of a healthier future—a bridge between the "having" of our current worldview and the deeper rhythms of life that transcend the material world and promote a better way of being.

We persist in feeling something underneath the surface of our material environment. Not only do we feel it, we need to express it in music, words, and dance. We have painted that feeling on the walls of caves and used it to serenade our children to sleep. It animates our sense of beauty and affinity with the environment and each other. Those that feel it most strongly steadfastly tell us that this energy is best expressed in the human acts of generosity, compassion, and humility. These qualities might seem to sit in a sharp contrast to the "selfishness" that some say is hardwired into our genetic makeup, but transcending, those unworthy qualities is exactly what the great spiritual leaders have counseled for centuries.

This is certainly not an invitation for useless guilt or self-recrimination. The central issue is if we can realize that what we do in our lives have effects that extend beyond the boundaries of personal horizon. This is the kind of maturity of being that has always been required of a just society and now occupies a position even more critical than in the past. In his criticism of the ineffectual liberalism of England before WWII, George Orwell wrote the following observation on the British Empire:

> **For apart from any other consideration, the high standard of life we enjoy in England depends upon our keeping a tight hold on the Empire. Under the capitalist system, in order that England may live in comparative comfort, a hundred million Indians must live on the verge of starvation—an evil state of affairs, but you acquiesce in it every time you step into a taxi or eat a plate of strawberries and cream.**

The same can be said of our present world. The empire of Britain, as with all empires, has vanished; but the present corporate empires exist on exactly the same principles. The megastore low prices on sneakers, clothes, or electronic gadgets still depend on someone living in squalid conditions and working for the better part of the day in order to eat. The system is broken and needs fixing. It only stands a chance of repair through awareness and action. All the usual seemingly rational hyperbole about how the poor have better money in the factory than before fly in the face of the real difference of being able to create food, shelter, and community that is self-sufficient as opposed to being the slave of foreign trade in dispensable trinkets.

What our more primitive hunter-gatherer and agricultural ancestors knew was that living in a way that enhances our being is best accomplished through cooperation. When we share, we not only enhance our own being but also express the best of our humanity. Giving unites us; greed separates us. Those axial teachers of human consciousness all taught that it was our ability to share that brought us most in line with our higher purpose. When we respect the needs of another as much as our own, we are aligning our energy with the power of the unknowable. If I am not mistaken, this is the Golden Rule.

Chapter Four

The Question of Consciousness

Breaking the Spell

As a species, we have a unique, marvelous, and dangerous gift—we can dream things. We can imagine the world different from what it is and change it. Our talent in this goes far beyond the capacity to survive. We can straighten rivers, and we can chop the tops off mountains. Skyscrapers and spaceships, new technologies and whole cities blink into and out of existence at our whim.

The creative impulse is a joy when used well. We can communicate a feeling with a poem, save labor with a plow, create a beautiful home to live in, or build a telescope to see the stars. Our imagination can widen our understanding, enhance our lives, and bring happiness. The same talent however can create machines of destruction and horror that kill in an instant and put cancer-causing chemicals in foods to give them a pleasing color to the eye.

Our thoughts and actions reflect the value we place on the whole process of life and our own place in that process. It matters little if the vision is formed by political, religious, or scientific belief. We are driven by a combination of experiences and concepts. If our concepts tell us that life is the result of a sequence of accidents in the chaos of a blind and soulless universe, those ideas will be reflected in our actions. If we believe that we are the creations of an angry and punishing god, the words and deeds will follow. Breaking this spell of our enchantments is not as easy as it might seem—simple yes, easy no.

Breaking the spell may require taking several giant steps backward from our present situation to find a different perspective. And yes, it means creating a new enchantment, one that is clearly aimed at going to the foundation of the life we share with a living planet. We will not have to go far since that vision already exists in many forms, but has a limited appeal since it always demands that we change on a fundamental level. It requires that we become conscious of our place in the scheme of things in a new way and that we reflect that way of being in our actions as well as our thoughts.

The good news is that we get to weave this new enchantment for ourselves and to weigh the benefits according to values that we deem essential for the health of ourselves, our children, and the web of life that we are part of.

A Macrobiotic Perspective

Understanding our own consciousness is a tricky business. It involves not only the process of being aware of what is going on around us but also the opinions, concepts, and feelings that influence that awareness. It deals with the experience as well as the enchantments; it involves our instinct as well as our intuition—our intellect and our inspiration. The relationship of all these facets of mind, body, and spirit provide the lens through which we perceive the world around us—perceptions that ultimately drive our actions.

In attempting to understand our behavior, every possible explanation has been put forward from genetic inheritance to childhood experience. Each school of thought has focused on finding a primary cause for the ways we convert the information we receive into the thoughts and actions that result. We are offered a smorgasbord of possibilities. We can choose from the position of the stars, original sin, survival mechanisms, potty training, a misaligned kundalini, faulty neural connections, or bad luck.

Many interesting schematic descriptions of how consciousness might evolve have been put forward as well. These models speak directly to the unfolding or development of consciousness. Some of these focus on spiritual growth as being the driving force behind the process. Some of the most interesting of them grow out of or reflect ideas put forward toward the beginning of the last century. The Indian writer, activist, yogi, and poet Sri Aurobindo and the French Jesuit priest, paleontologist, and philosopher Teilhard de Chardin both put forward a vision of conscious evolution leading to spiritual awakening. It is within this tradition that George Ohsawa developed his macrobiotic philosophy.

Ohsawa saw himself as a bridge between Asia and the West, bringing the samurai code of his own ancestry into the world of modern materialistic thought. He came to feel that scientific materialism, particularly medicine, was following a shortsighted path. He saw the growth of Western medicine as a direct threat to the capacity of individuals to manage their own health, making them slaves to a system that was only concerned with symptomatic treatment of sickness and silent about prevention. Taking a page from the Taoist sages of ancient China, he promoted self-discipline and awareness as a path to health and freedom.

Ohsawa's idea of freedom began with physical health and specifically the ability to control health through dietary principles. From that simple foundation, he enlarged this idea to include a wide range of social and spiritual influences. It was his statements on diet that received the most attention, often to the neglect of the broader scope of his philosophy. Similar to the American psychologist Abraham Maslow, Ohsawa saw consciousness developing through a layering of specific human needs.

In describing the outward progression toward what I have called the authentic self, Ohsawa acknowledged the relationship between the physical and the emotional, the ideological and the spiritual. He showed how each of these elements were related to the issue of health in the most comprehensive sense. He pictured this as a spiral expanding out from the innate potential of the embryo. As we move through infancy, childhood, adolescence, and onward, we incorporate our physical, emotional, social, and environmental experience into our being.

The physical, emotional, and cultural influences that surround us become the foundation of our beliefs and form the focus of the lens through which we see the world. This filtered vision shows us how the world works and our place in it. The problem lies in the fact that all to often we become entangled in one phase of that development, and it becomes the dominant feature in our point of view. We have a natural drive toward realizing our full potential, but if the more basic human needs are not met, it is difficult to move toward that goal.

In this single sense, his model is similar to Maslow's hierarchy of needs. Each arena of experience contains an element that is essential for our full development. This model is helpful in understanding the relationship between physical, emotional, and spiritual health as long as we understand that it is not a strictly linear process. While the dynamics of this pattern can be accelerated or contravened by illness, shock, or a moment of ecstasy, the basic needs stay the same.

Maslow was unique in that his focus was on the healthy psyche as opposed to mental illness. He saw the basic urge for what he termed as self-actualization as the driving force of a happy life. Both Ohsawa and Maslow had a clear vision of human development progressing from physical and emotional fulfillment outward from the self to broader concerns of social harmony and justice, leading to the peak experiences of love, happiness, and fulfillment. Ohsawa's work was greatly influenced by Oriental medicine and so focused on the impact of biological integrity and its effect on this process.

Biology and Awareness

The first two areas of development have to do with the drive to exist and to experience pleasure. Discussions of consciousness that do not take into account the role of physical functioning are shortsighted at best. Our experience of ourselves coupled with our sensitivity to our environment forms the foundation of our attitudes toward the world we live in. We can see the first level of development as being an analogy of the driving force of DNA. We know about the spiral dance of yin and yang described by the attraction of sperm to egg that leads to the great mystery of life. When seen under a microscope, we can almost feel the quivering magnetic pull of these carriers of life as they are drawn together. It is a drama with the most profound consequences.

Upon the meeting of sperm and egg, an explosive multiplication of cells occurs, which transforms the single cell of the egg into a vibrant collection of millions of cells within weeks. By the time the embryo is only eight weeks old, there are recognizable features of hands and feet, tiny eyes and mouth, and the spirit energy of the heart throbs, marking the rhythm of life within.

All of this process happens within the inner ocean of the mother's body. It is nourished by the soil of the flesh, watered by the supporting inner sea of the womb, and bathed in the rhythm of life—the drumbeat of the mother heart, the coursing of blood through vessels, and the rocking of the movement of the mother's body. The growth that takes place lays down the systems and structures of a complete human form and builds in the potentials that mark our kind. The womb is the universe that supports this growth, yielding to the needs of the growing life it contains. The mother, a small version of Gaia, supports the emerging life in the same way, the planet supports humankind.

This is one of the most important periods in our life. It is here where the seeds of potential are formed. The unique focus in human development is concentrated in the brain and nervous system. This is the site where the great leap of form takes place, creating an organ of perception, reflection, and action of astounding capacity.

The massive biological change and development that happens in such a brief period of time is almost beyond comprehension. The nine-month period of gestation is the biological equivalent of over three billion years of evolution. Every day is a represents thousands of years of cellular development and organization. Assigning consciousness to this process might be argued, but the fact is that all life-forms have a consciousness in some degree. A flower responds to sun by opening or closing, animals respond to their environments. We have come to ascribe consciousness only to those human attributes of thinking or conceptualizing—a great mistake if we are to understand the world we live in.

Once set in motion, the mechanics of this process will continue till the moment of our death. It is represented not only in the minute behavior of individual cells but also in the autonomic nervous system. Taken as a whole, this process represents the body's desire to stay alive. Our drive toward water, food and air as well as our sexual drive and our innate need to feel safe are part of this vital expression of living.

The Chinese saw that this physical development reflected certain energetic qualities of the parents. The Chi (energy) of the parents are combined with the physical nourishment of the embryo to influence the constitution or energetic qualities of the child. This constitutional energy described certain tendencies that would manifest as the child developed. Some would be more attracted to action, some more passive, some would be more influenced by their intellect, and some by emotion. These qualities need not be seen as a command but rather as a pull in a particular direction.

While we have no control over this period of our development, we can maximize the gifts we are given. This is clearly evident in men and women who were disabled and compensated by developing other aspects of their physical, emotional, or spiritual being. When faced with their spirit to rise above their challenges, it makes most of the trials of daily life seem trivial. Personal development is focused on stimulating or recovering as much as possible our biological potential. The roots of our authentic self lie within our biology. Without roots, no branch; no branch, no leaf; no leaf, no flower. This internal world of our physical environment is initially led outward to its flowering by the senses.

The reactive qualities of the nervous system develop quite early. The skin surface of the developing fetus has sensitivity to changes in its immediate environment and reacts to them. This peripheral sensitivity becomes increasingly acute to the point where sound vibration can be received through the amniotic fluid, producing a variety of reactions such as abrupt movements, kicking of the feet, or clenching of the hands. If the first stages of development are aimed at creating the organic foundation for our internal functioning, the sense organs give us the capacity to engage with the environment that lies outside our physical boundaries.

After birth, the child begins a period of experimentation that stimulates the sense organs. An increased sophistication of the child's ability to receive and interpret sensory information grows out from them, expanding the perimeters of their world. The senses of touch, taste, and smell, the more primitive of senses, seem to develop more acutely during the first phases, followed by the development of hearing and, finally, sight. It is interesting to note that sensory perception developing along these lines moves increasingly out and away from the body. We grow out into the world.

Through the development of the senses, the child is discovering a separate identity, one that is not directly physically connected to another individual. The interaction between the child and its environment is of primary importance. An environment that is either deficient in appropriate sensory stimuli or overloaded with a chaotic flow of information can be traumatic.

It is necessary for the child to feel confident and secure within its environment so that new or unusual information is not perceived as threatening but rather is approached with curiosity. It has been shown that exposure to nature can be an important key to the development of physical and emotional health. This should not be surprising since our senses are most finely tuned to the working of the life force through the medium of the natural world. The sounds, sights, and smells of nature speak directly to the biological and energetic rhythms of our own bodies. People go to the seashore or the mountains to recharge themselves; they take a walk in the park to calm their minds. The senses are a basic portal into the workings of Gaia and to our connection to her.

As the modern environment becomes dominated by the mind and hand of man, the experience of nature becomes more alien. Many people are frightened by the experience of nature or find it too placid. The ability to be spiritually uplifted by music or birdsong, to savor a healthy meal or clean water, to register the affection in a lover's touch can wither without nourishment. The more that the senses are overwhelmed by the relentless static that characterizes the built spaces, the more dull they become to the subtleties of natural process. We can easily lose the ability to discern the difference between what serves us and what we should avoid.

The terms *emotions* and *feelings* are often used interchangeably. We say we "feel" sad or happy, depressed or positive; this may be because what we term as emotions are extensions of the senses and intimately associated with them. Emotions elicit physical responses, changes in heart rate, breathing, and body temperature among them. The opposite is also true; physical sensations are powerful emotional triggers. I will revisit his connection between emotion and physical condition in later chapters.

As we explore the realm of the senses, one distinction becomes apparent: there are aspects of the environment that respond back to us. The people in our life show us cause and effect in a very direct way. As powers of perception become more acute, we begin to see faces, bodies and hear voices of those of our own kind who respond to our movements and sounds. This give-and-take of sound, touch, and movements lays the cornerstone for our first communication. How the people and events around us bring pleasure or pain is the bedrock of our emotional landscape.

Culture and Consciousness

The next stage in the development of our consciousness is dominated by emotions, concepts, and ideals. This arena of activity contains the influence of family, language, and formation of belief. The first two stages of biological development describe the structure of our physical being. Our family and cultural world are the primary influences on the formation of our emotional and intellectual landscape.

The level of interaction we have with our parents or other humans who come into our range of sensitivity are of a special kind. The smells of our mother can be determined in the early days of life as distinct from the smell of someone else; we learn to distinguish the sound of familiar voices and all the impressions that accompany them. Much of what is identified as emotion, at this early age, stems from a desire for physical pleasure, safety, and comfort. In early stages of infant development, a child will express emotional response at the sight of its mother, but of course, the mother in most cases is the source of physical pleasure since she is supplying food, warmth, and security. As we develop other types of interactions, we begin to include more than the maternal. Our desire for sensory satisfaction slowly move out into the more subtle areas of comfort, security, friendship, and acknowledgment. It is fair to say that emotional communication is our first language.

A child learns how to communicate what he or she wants from others through body language, facial expression, and vocalizing. The emotional sensations we develop begin to color and enhance our experience. The fulfillment being sought is still personal pleasure, but we also learn that we can stimulate pleasure or arouse anger in others through the energy of our emotions. We are constantly observing the actions of those around us to learn how to use our feelings to communicate our needs and desires as well as what behavior is approved or disapproved. We are learning what works and what doesn't work.

We are exploring an emotional landscape that is being largely defined by the immediate family. It is a landscape defined by subtleties of expression. The lessons we learn and those around us largely dictate the areas of experience we explore. These explorations may be joyous and exciting or frightening and painful. We develop the capacity to know when "something is wrong." The slope of shoulder or the turn of the mouth can communicate volumes of information. We learn to interpret the emotional states of others through these signs. Our emotional vocabulary provides the foundation for much of our internal narrative.

Are the boundaries placed on our emotional life filled with love, encouragement, and self-empowerment, or are we constrained in our behavior, sternly judged, or abused? We learn at an early age what emotions bring results and which are wasted. The emotions are a "stirring up" of the feelings and an excitation of our life force energy. They will greatly impact the ways in which we express our own dreams and visions and the degree of comfort we have in expressing our inner self. This emotional education has a tendency to formalize in our body as well as our mind.

If the family and early social interactions color our emotional experience, it is our culture that provides the organizing principles. Part of being human is the desire to know how things work. All this effort into making things fit can be hard work. Politics, science, religion, philosophy, all the enchantments described in the first chapter are a reflection of this desire. When those organizing principles lead us into a larger curiosity and experience of life, it is education; when it constricts our vision, it is indoctrination. The rigidity of conceptual models can produce a correspondent rigidity in the growing child or lay down the seeds for rebellion if the rigidity of the models flies in the face of experienced reality. A ready example of this is found in the confusion often caused in children through contradictions between what has been taught as a moral precept and actions that seem to be socially acceptable. A child may be told that lying is wrong and even be punished for telling a lie and yet observe an acceptance of it between adults.

We are told why certain things must be done, what works and what doesn't, and a wide range of ideas that we have no way of testing through our own experience. We are certainly told about the significance or value of things. The mind organizes the information that we receive through our senses and filtered through our emotions according to these guidelines. These concepts are the glue that holds together our interaction with our particular tribe. It is concepts, not blood, that binds cultures.

We are learning about life from the moment of conception. Our moral, religious, and intellectual training invariably aim us down a narrow path of what is accepted as true and valuable. Adults, figures of authority, and experience present these concepts to us. The coupling of emotion and concept is a powerful concoction. When concepts are driven by emotional force, they become powerful tools for control and manipulation.

The communication of ideas in modern society have become dependent on emotional "spin." Information has become a product to be sold rather that a thought to be shared. Television, newspapers, and magazines rely increasingly on emotional impact to engage the consumer in a way that is less thoughtful and more thrilling. The exact same event or piece of research or new idea is shaped in hundreds of ways to appeal to the emotional bias of the reader or viewer and tailored to benefit the goals of an institution or an item for consumption.

This approach is reflected in early schooling in Western societies with the increased reliance of television as a "teaching aid." The medium itself does not allow time for thought or introspection but puts teaching into the field of entertainment and perilously close to indoctrination or propaganda. This is further complicated when we place religious dogma into the mix. The approach to teaching (at home or in school) that indoctrinates is counter to the development of wisdom. Wisdom depends on experience and the ability to exercise the intuitive faculties of the mind. Societies suffer when wisdom is not valued. Wisdom gives the ability to think in a holistic manner, to bridge apparent separations.

Social development requires the ability of the individual to identify and experience being part of a social unit as well as to openly and safely question it. It has to do with an actual sensation of connectedness between individuals, being part of the same underlying continuum of energy. If the conceptual and emotional environment of the community nourishes the healthy integration of this process, it is a stepping-stone for a vibrant and healthy society.

Many of the ideologies of the modern world are built on basic concepts that are not discussed. What if our religious theology is based on fears of what might happen to us when we die or our political ideologies are rationalizations for protecting our wealth? In these cases, it is really the emotions of fear of death or the security implied in wealth that are ennobled by having a broader notion that they can nestle into. Narrow visions of religious faith or patriotic zeal are often represented as well-reasoned theories when in fact they are pandering to emotional insecurities.

Spiritual Ecology

A person with evolved consciousness experiences all of the influences mentioned above with one important distinction—they are not obsessed by or attached to any of them. The body is nurtured and cared for, but without attachment; sensory information is enjoyed deeply, but does not rule action. Emotions are felt, but not used as a sole basis for judgment or as a means of manipulation. Concepts are used dynamically without need of dogma. Social decisions are nurtured with long-term effect and the next generation considered. Ideology is aligned with an appreciation of nature and respect for all living things. The development of this view unsurprisingly connects one with the creative forces that guide the rhythms of life. It involves experiencing the world in a new way. It is a way of being that holds a vibrant and uplifting vision of the world but is capable of the engagement with the mundane without losing that vision.

I am reminded of a Zen story about two monks who make a vow to avoid contact with women as part of their training. As they set out on a journey, they come to a river that is swollen by the rains. On the bank of the river stands a beautiful woman who cannot cross. The first monk scurries past her, fords the river, and turns to wait for his companion. He is shocked to see that the second monk has the woman on his back and is carrying her across.

As they continue up the road, the first monk is obviously angry and upset. His friend finally asks him why he is distressed, and the monk replies that he cannot believe that his companion has broken a vow so quickly. "You carried her across, she was hanging on to you." In response, the second monk replies, "Yes, I carried her across the river, but I sat her down miles ago, you are still carrying her."

Even though we may suffer hardships, sickness, or despair, our spiritual essence is there as long as we live. We may have areas of our lives that have not been fully nourished, but we can rise above them all by accepting the challenge of change. It is our habits that hold us back, habits of thought, action, and emotion. It is easy to consign these habits to fate or bad luck or punishment to be endured, but if we have the clarity to see them as aberrations of our real potential, we have the capacity to change them. We often miss the opportunity to transform our life simply because we hold back from the first step. That first step does not need to be something complex; it can be simple and still be effective. The difficulties we face usually arise from the resistance to change the physical, emotional, and cultural addictions to our behavior.

Chapter Five

Health and Sickness

Embracing Life

Our modern understanding of health is drowning in a sea of information that weighs us down rather than lifts us up. Rather than pursuing health in order to live our lives more abundantly and to develop our human potential, we have turned it into a response to our fear of death, sickness, or an unattractive appearance. A quick scanning of the news in any week is enough to establish that health is a major issue within Western culture. Magazines, newspapers, television programs, and books mark the swings between the fascination, confusion, obsession, and fear that the topic pulls to surface. Much of the confusion has to do with the simple fact that the matter of our health has been complicated beyond normal understanding. We are bombarded with conflicting information from supposedly reliable sources. We hear about diets to make us thinner, supplements to improve our brain function, vitamins to cure cancer, and the newest celebrity exercise craze guaranteed to extend our lives.

This is all set against the background of medical and pharmaceutical advancements to repair that dodgy heart or surgically remove those pesky bags under our eyes or magically increase our sexual vitality. There is always some kind of science that is touted as proof that the technique is safe, effective, and guaranteed to work. The uncomfortable fact is that the most reliable information shows that what we eat and the way we live are the causes of our most common health problems.

None of this is new. Most of the connections between our daily habits and disease have been known for decades. The information rises to the surface every few years and then sinks like a stone, lying dormant till the tides change. Our memories are short in these matters. When it rises once again into the light, it is classified under the heading of "Things We Really Should Do Something About." One of the primary reasons for confusion in matters of health is that we have no real definition of what health is.

Outside of the more cosmetic issues of how young we look or the lack of any irritating discomfort or bad news from a blood test, we have no standard of judging our health levels. We need to establish a definition of health that goes beyond the mere treatment of symptoms and returns common sense to the health debate. Our ideas regarding health are a defining issue as to who we are in the world, our attitudes about life and death, and our respect for the process of creation.

We may eat a terrible diet, smoke or drink to excess, or form demeaning relationships, all with awareness that something is wrong, but seemingly unable to shift course. There are many possible answers to the "Why do I do it?" question. The connecting thread to most of these answers is that while we may be able to make out a possible cause for a problem, changing it lays outside our immediate control. We have given up control of our lives and simply don't believe we can get it back. This erosion of personal power often results from the lack of a clear sense of direction capable of informing our actions, combined with a developed sense of personal power to act effectively.

Health describes not only our internal state of being but also how we express that state of being in thought and action. When we say that a person has a "healthy attitude" or develops "healthy relationships" or is blessed with a "healthy curiosity," these statements speak to our recognition how health is reflected in our daily behavior. There are definite indications of good health that go beyond the lack of discomfort or pain. Looking for the qualities of health in our daily routine can provide us with useful benchmarks. Two road maps to understanding health that we have inherited in macrobiotic thinking are Ohsawa's descriptions of health and sickness.

His vision of health is balanced by a description of how sickness develops in a systematic way. This genesis of sickness is helpful in providing a way of understanding the interaction of various physical and emotional factors that lead to illness. This model also provides a means for simple self-assessment. While Ohsawa's ideas are built around the physical origins of all sickness, I have broadened the scope of possible cause. In later chapters, I have taken some liberties with his original definitions.

The Qualities of Health

Vitality of Thought and Action: The authentic self is capable of quick decisive action in both work and play. This vitality is a reflection of the life process, a process of forward momentum. The authentic self moves forward toward the realization of life purpose, dreams, and visions. This forward momentum may be sidetracked, blocked, or diverted for a period of time; but it always returns to its true course of action. When a child or even a household pet is lethargic, we worry about them; we recognize the lethargy as an indicator of imbalance. Increasingly, both adults and children complain that they are exhausted, worn out, and stressed. We have come to accept this lack of energy as normal. If you think of the people admired in the world, they will invariably be men and women who have a zest for life. Even if faced with difficulty, they are capable of rising to the occasion.

An Appetite for Life: Our existence is dependent on what we take in, and a healthy appetite is a sign of good health. We are constantly nurtured by the world around us. This nourishment comes from nature directly and through the food we eat as well as the information and emotional messages we receive from culture and personal relationships. All that we take in is information for the body, mind, and spirit to process. The quality of this consumption can either nourish or stifle our quest for health. Sometimes the appetite for life is deflected or stifled by the objects of our desire. A good appetite for life means that we nourish the authentic self and not the habits that hold us in sickness and confusion. To survive, to prosper, and to develop healthy appetites, it is essential that we develop discernment.

Discernment has to do with making healthy choices and developing healthy habits because they make you feel good, not because you feel you have to. Too often, a healthy habit is pursued because of a moral or intellectual impulse. This can lead to dogmatic thinking, unhappiness, and even poor physical results. Discipline is fine as a starting point, but the goal is freedom. Discernment does not have to do with a moral code. When our appetites and our health are in alignment, we desire that which serves our purpose—we crave what is good for us. As discernment develops, it becomes spontaneous.

Having healthy appetites does not mean that our actions are predictable or boring. When we have experienced positive outcomes from developing healthy habits, the occasional diversion from the norm can be experienced as an adventure, not a trap. Living a life that is rich in cultural diversity, physical pleasure, and creative activity should be part of a healthy life. Health is not characterized by a retreat from society but a vibrant engagement with it.

Relaxation and Sleep: Emotional and physical stress have become primary issues in modern health care. Stress is now listed along with diet as a contributing factor in the development of most degenerative diseases. Deep and restful sleep is indication of good health. The body requires good sleep in order to rebuild the immune system and to release physical and emotional tension in the body. Sleep is the natural antidote to stress. Good sleep is built on the ability for the body to move into a state of restfulness and then repeat a number of full sleep cycles. Each time we move through a full cycle, a new depth of relaxation and release is reached. If we are not sleeping well, our system becomes compromised, and we lose vitality. When we have experienced deep and regenerative sleep, we wake up refreshed and ready to begin the day.

Good sleep is also productive of meaningful dreaming. Meaningful dreams resonate with the authentic self; they often contain instructions for future action, symbolic reference to qualities we need to nourish in our lives, or provide supportive lessons for our development. They are memorable, detailed, and provide a poetic vision of the important issues in our lives that takes us beyond our analytical waking behavior.

Good sleep is complemented by the ability to relax and be mindful in any surrounding. This quality of the body and mind allows us to be quiet and restful so that we can better experience the present moment. The ability to relax is essential in today's society where the pace of living is often hectic and can easily distract us or force us to tune out our surroundings.

Good Memory: Good memory is associated with good sleep. When we are in the deepest sleep, the mind has the capacity to organize the experiences of the day for future reference. The authentic self has access to the past in order to inform future vision and present action. The memory of the authentic self goes beyond individual experience. Our cellular memory contains within it recollection of our collective past and allows us to better interpret the dreams and visions we have. The psychologist Carl Jung referred to this kind of memory as the collective unconsciousness. For me, this quality of memory seems essential since it allows us to better understand the symbolic nature of folk wisdom, mythology, and historical fact with deeper appreciation.

Good Humor: Life is filled with paradox, change, and the unexpected. How we respond to these twists and turns is a reflection of our adaptability. An appreciation of the unpredictable and the illogical is a reflection of our sense of humor. This is especially true in our capacity to laugh at ourselves. Even when we are pursuing a noble cause, we should be able to find amusement in our serious intent. The authentic self is aware of the transient nature of life. Everything comes to an end. Full engagement means that we play the game of life to its fullest, knowing that the universe moves on long after we are gone, and our personal plans and schemes have been forgotten.

Clarity of Thought and Action: When we are experiencing health, our reactions are not only quick but also appropriate. I was once in a restaurant where a tableside preparation went wrong, and the table and the side tray burst into flames. From my side of the room, it looked like total panic. People jumped from their tables, knocking dishes to the floor, waiters ran into each other, and a state of pandemonium took over.

In the middle of the confusion, I saw one man, from several tables away, purposely walk to the service area. He calmly picked up a jug of water and made his way through the crowd. He ceremoniously poured the water over the flaming mess, took wet napkins off the table, and dampened the fire. The fire was out when the waiters emerged from the kitchen with the extinguishers. When he was done, he returned to his table, sat down, and continued his meal. I felt like applauding. The ability to act decisively does not mean that we are being impetuous. Sometimes the best course is to avoid action. Knowing the difference between rash and responsible action is a challenge that requires self-reflection and a dispassionate assessment of the effect of what we do.

Appreciation of Nature: We are part of a living planet that is a reflection of natural process. Nature is both the source of our being and our home. It is the tangible representation of the Tao, the unknowable energy of creation. When we pay attention to the order of natural process and apply its lessons in our lives, we are rewarded by health and increased authenticity of being. The authentic self is drawn to the rhythms and cycles of change so that the individual life serves the whole.

A healthy person recognizes the natural environment as sacred space. The concepts of ecological living and environmental justice come naturally when we are healthy. This is reflected in the life choices we make from the foods we eat to the economy of our homes. The authentic self loves nature and delights in being close to it. When isolation from nature dominates and we live in the world of the built space with no exit and no skills to bring nature into our lives, we suffer. That suffering is labeled as stress.

Stress and Modern Living

Stress is what is experienced when any system is exposed to forces that challenge its integrity. Much of modern life is founded on ideas that do not take into account the health and welfare of the individual. From the design of our cities to the content of our education, we have developed a culture in which the most important qualities of human life are expendable. Much of this is done in the name of progress and economic benefit.

Stress manifests in a number of ways. Among the most common are nutritional stress, anatomical stress, emotional stress, and environmental stress. Each of these has profound influences on our health, and most can be reduced or eliminated through simple methods that are discussed in the following chapters. When experienced together, they produce many of the maladies that are common in our society from cancer to mental disorders. They often confound medical science and confuse the ill since there is no single causal factor. The real solution is most often a dramatic shift in lifestyle—a path seldom taken.

Nutritional stress is the starting point for any macrobiotic discussion. It is the result of taking in foods that are inappropriate for human consumption. That is a very simple concept that keeps being put to the side of the endless debates on diet and nutrition. Many of the foods we eat are simply toxic in nature or in the way they are used. They include chemical additives, foods with little nutritional value, foods that are not suited for our individual energy needs, foods that are not suited for our environment, or foods that challenge our individual state of health. Because these foods are not naturally suited for us, they produce stress.

The body is designed to produce health; it will try to accommodate the poor choices we make, laboring under the burden of poor judgment. Our addiction to poor nutrition guarantees a toxic condition, making us vulnerable to degenerative process and opportunistic infection. It also directly affects our sensitivity to our own physical condition and our state of mind.

Anatomical stress is provoked by static patterns of physical movement and a sedentary way of living. Standing all day on concrete floors or hunched over a computer terminal or spending most of our time seated places unrelenting pressure on joints and muscles. This type of activity can become formalized into muscle tension if not corrected through other types of movement or exercise.

Tension that is held in the body for prolonged periods affects the flow of energy, blood, and lymph and can lead to more serious problems. The key to avoiding this kind of stress is good nutrition and increased movement, especially movement that stretches and invigorates the body.

Emotional stress on the development of sickness has drawn increased interest over the past twenty years. It is now generally agreed that certain individuals internalize emotional conflict in ways that can do profound physical damage. As more is learned about the working of the human brain, it is obvious that mental confusion, fear, and suppressed anger can provoke changes in blood chemistry and even in the functioning of the immune system. What is not really addressed is why some people can deal with emotional turmoil in ways that are nondestructive and others, when faced with a similar challenge, are devastated.

Part of the answer to this question may lie in the little known effect of the opposite side of the coin. What is the role of physical health in the development of our emotional life. In a later chapter I will discuss the way that Chinese medicine may provide valuable insight. By linking both the internal and external influences on our emotional patterns we can come to a more complete understanding of the body-mind relationship.

Environmental stress describes our response to the built environment. The effects of urban environments on health attract increasing attention by health professionals. This very broad category includes a number of factors. The most obvious offenders are the toxic compounds that are released into the air we breathe and the water we drink. Along with the appearance of chemicals in the food chain and the addition of chemicals used in food manufacture, they comprise a powerful cocktail of poisonous substances that are absorbed daily by most of the population. The fact that many of these chemicals cause cellular mutation should be a cause for great concern.

The Stages of Imbalance

Ohsawa's description of a progressive development of sickness is an interesting model for reflection. The main element here is the understanding that with the exception of accidents or birth defects, illness does not simply drop from the sky.

There are symptoms that are often ignored because they are deemed normal or marginal when in fact they may be significant indicators of a deeper problem. Coupled with this is the seemingly obvious insight that the systems of the body are part of a whole. This fact is often ignored completely in modern health care.

Tiredness: Lack of vitality is a preliminary symptom in the process of sickness. When there is not enough energy for normal movement or the lack of vitality and enthusiasm in dealing with day-to-day life, it is a problem that needs attention. Biologically this may be a result of imbalances in the digestive and excretory systems. If the intestinal environment is not healthy, toxicity builds up. If the abuse is continued, it is absorbed into the bloodstream, putting stress on the kidneys and the liver.

When animals or young children experience these symptoms, their normal response is to sleep and to reject food. This allows the body to rest and usually corrects any temporary imbalance; it is a natural reaction to these symptoms. When a child becomes lethargic, friends and parents become worried and see this as an important symptom. When an adult becomes tired, we rationalize it in hundreds of ways. The primary reason put forth is that our work is too hard when in fact we labor much less than our ancestors. Coffee and other caffeinated beverages, simple sugars, and medication are often used to mask the underlying symptoms. Since it is assumed that modern living wears you out, this important symptom is neglected. Exercise and simple dietary improvements are often rejected because the person is too tired to pursue them. This rationale is curious since most of the people I have counseled on health experience increased energy when they introduce these simple acts into their lives.

Physical Inflexibility: If the level of toxicity produced by inappropriate nutrition and poor digestive function is allowed to continue, then symptoms move to the next stage of development. This is typified by lack of mobility in the joints of the body or stiffness and tension in the muscles. In this case, natural toxic by-products in the areas surrounding the joints and in the muscles cannot be adequately transported for excretion due to the rise of toxicity in the blood.

In its beginning stages, this imbalance can usually be dealt with easily by correcting diet and using appropriate exercise. Adults very seldom perceive stiffness or constraints on mobility to be important unless associated with persistent pain. The causes for these problems are normally ascribed to such things as aging, the wrong shoes, or a mattress that is either too soft or too hard.

Rigid movements and the disappearance of our native agility and quickness of response are seen to be part and parcel of the general tragedy of existence. Many will seek out massage or spinal adjustment here, but if there are no changes in personal lifestyle, the problems will return. I have had clients who were in their thirties tell me that persistent muscle or joint pain was simply because they were getting old! Pain medication is used by a vast majority of the population, further suppressing the symptoms, ignoring the root cause of the problem and accepting a life of limited activity.

Toxicity of the Blood: When toxic levels in the bloodstream have not been redressed, we develop what Ohsawa called sickness of the blood. The symptoms of illness at this level are peripheral enough to cause the individual little or no concern in many cases. At this stage in the development of illness, the excretory functions of the skin come into play. Symptoms at this level manifest themselves most usually in changes of skin tone, texture or color, and/or excessive sensitivity or irritation of the skin or mucous membranes.

The term commonly used in macrobiotics and some other forms of alternative health care is *discharge*. The body is attempting to throw off toxicity in an attempt to redress the internal balance and harmony of the body's chemistry. Pimples, boils, puffiness of the face, discharge of mucus, excessive tearing of the eyes, or accumulation of waxy buildup in the ears are the basic qualities of a Shakespearian curse, are all common symptoms of this stage. In modern medicine, treatment for these symptoms is usually some form of suppression.

If we have a running nose, diarrhea, fever, or persistent acne, we do everything possible to inhibit the natural rebalancing of the body to run its course. This is often done for reasons of convenience or cosmetic considerations without regard to the cause. As in the above stages of illness, the body is continually sending us messages to adjust the course of our actions. We not only have lost the ability to acknowledge this simple fact, we are encouraged to ignore these important communications. This process of suppression of symptom denies us the ability to truly understand how our body works and to explore ways to establish self-mastery.

Emotional Vulnerability: There is a direct relationship between the general well-being of the body and the building up of emotional tension. If the body is in a dynamic state of balanced health, then coping with external influences happens with a greater degree of ease. When the body is ill at ease, external influences become irritants that promote the holding of tension within the body. When we suffer from this held tension, stress is increased. Stress naturally seeks release. Pent-up anger, frustration or grief begin to erupt with little or no provocation. The important factors are where and how tension is held, the biological origin of the tension, and the kind of external stimulus needed for its release.

In studying human behavior, we ascribe values to this process of release that are often arbitrary and subjective. The body's primitive reactive nature seeks to discharge energy that is stagnant or irritating. The release can actually have a temporary cleansing consequence. This is why after "letting go" of anger, having a good cry, or any other kind of physical release of emotional tension can produce a state of relaxation and clearheadedness.

This does not mean that all emotional distress is caused by what we eat or a physical imbalance. It is simply an acknowledgment that the role of diet, exercise, and other simple lifestyle changes can have a positive influence on changing the emotional landscape. It also points to the possibility that our physical condition can predicate us toward particular emotional behavior. A more detailed look at some of the correlations between emotion and physical condition are discussed in later chapters.

Degenerative Process: The first four stages of developing illness all involve an attempt on the part of the body to discharge toxicity and tension and to create better balance. If the symptoms are not reversed in the prior levels, then the stage is set for degenerative process. The chemistry of the blood will have by this time become chronically altered, and the tissues of the body become increasingly rigid. Circulation and normal metabolism are interrupted. The body begins to lose its biological integrity, tissue begins to degenerate or mutate, and more serious or life-threatening processes begin.

These processes do not happen overnight but are the outcome of years of neglect. If the early stages of illness do not raise an alarm through the severity of the symptoms, they often pass unnoticed. Symptoms at this level can develop for years before they are diagnosed by conventional means. By the time that the symptoms become chronic or debilitating, they invite more aggressive medical intervention. When tiredness becomes overwhelming, when stiffness morphs into arthritis or chronic back pain, or emotional imbalance threatens social interaction, the level of treatment escalates. This is where most individuals give away complete control of their bodies to the institutions of medicine or psychiatry. This is where the most potent pharmaceuticals come to bear and where the body's natural healing capacities are most strongly suppressed and compromised.

Dysfunction of the Nervous System: Macrobiotic thinking has long held that the degenerative process compromises the function of the nervous system. The brain and nervous system are especially sensitive to changes in blood chemistry. The more primitive parts of the brain, those dealing with the most basic biological functions of the body, have precedence when the body is in a state of imbalance. This is recognized relative to extreme dysfunctions of the body where the patient may experience dementia, slip into a coma, or become delirious.

The symptoms on this extreme level are characterized by a diminished ability to accurately perceive our relationship with the world around us, persistent irritation, depression, anxiety, etc., or unusual nervous habits. When we are extremely imbalanced, our attention is drawn back to ourselves. We become self-centered. This can be seen as a protective impulse. As the body becomes weaker and disease processes becomes entrenched, the attention of the organism is drawn back to itself. One of the attributes of health is a curiosity and desire to explore the environment. When biological instability develops, this process is reversed. We are prone to rationalize the way we feel and the way we act in ways that are self-serving. We are seeing the world through the veil of our condition.

Isolation: In chapter 2, I discussed the softening of personal boundaries as an aspect of the authentic self; this stage of imbalance is the exact opposite. This is the most debilitating process in human life. As our attention is drawn back to ourselves and held there, we begin to separate, to withdraw from the world surrounding us. Our life patterns become repetitious; we become caught in a cage of our own unwitting design. Either a perceived inability to change or an adamant resistance to doing so characterizes this self-entrapment. Statements like "I'm too weak," "I can't change," or "I don't understand" are characteristic of the perceived inability to change. The latter by "I won't change" or "I don't need to change." Both attitudes are simply different sides of the same coin. The personal narrative is locked into place and is either a story of Me against the World or the World against Me.

The good news is that we can unravel this web and find our true path. The battle for the authentic self is waged against the fortress of learned behavior, habit, and a defiant worldview. When we embrace change and are willing to learn from nature, a new way of seeing emerges. George Ohsawa called it putting on the Magic Spectacles. It is a transformative way of living and leads to an enhanced experience of our own authenticity.

Chapter Six

Lessons of Wind and Water

Life Experience and Energy

We live in a culture where the analytical use of language rules supreme. We expect a certain precision in the description of everything from nutrition to physiology even when we are accepting that description as an act of faith. The assurance that we will get enough protein from a particular food or that we have a genetic disposition to develop a particular disease impresses us even if we have only the foggiest idea what a gene is or where a protein lives when it's not in a hamburger. Science is the dominant force in our understanding of the physical world. The language of science is a powerful incantation. The only problem with this is that very few of us live with an awareness of microscopic detail. Most human beings live in the realm of feelings. The fact that feelings are not easy to analyze does nothing to undermine their importance. This is not to say that feeling is superior to thinking either. Both are need to be integrated for the authentic self to thrive. Intuition, instinct, insight, and precognition are "felt" rather than "thought."

One of the problems in understanding ancient philosophies or medicine has to do with language. The languages of tribal peoples are most often filled with metaphor and poetry. The descriptions of physical, emotional, or spiritual states are filled with reference to natural phenomena such as wind, water, or the cycles of the seasons. They often refer to qualities of emotion or animal behavior. It is not uncommon to ascribe plant or animal characteristics to human conditions. This is a language based on feeling states—the language of sensory experience and imagination. It speaks to the energy that unites the viewer with the view. While the language of science is excellent for discussing the material detail of nature and the separation between the warp and the woof, the poetic language of the past allows us to see the complete fabric with the design revealed. The most consistent view of the patterns of nature have to do with the dance of opposites expressed in China and Japan as yin and yang.

We are all used to the folk wisdom that life progresses in cycles. "After the rain comes the rainbow" or "life has its ups and downs" or "after the darkness comes the dawn"—our language is filled with references to the fact that nothing in life moves in a straight line. Even our study of human history shows the cyclic rise and fall of empires. This movement is evident in nature as the movement of sap to the branches in summer and the roots in winter or the yearly migration patterns of birds.

The appreciation of this flux and flow of Spirit lies at the foundation of a powerful source of wisdom. Listen to what two different men with wisdom have to say about yin and yang. The first are the words attributed to Jesus in the scriptures called the Nag Hammadi Library. This unique collection of ancient volumes was discovered in 1945 and is thought by many scholars to be the writings of an early Gnostic Christian community from about AD 140. The section called the Gospel of Thomas is interesting because the words attributed to Jesus contain many stories found in the Bible, but some with a distinctly different tone from the stories as they were translated from later sources.

> **Jesus said to them—"When you make the two one, and when you make the inner as the outer and the outer as the inner and the above as the below, and when you make the male and the female into a single one, so that the male will not be male and the female not be female, when you make eyes in the place of an eye, and a hand in the place of a hand, and the foot in the place of a foot, and an image in the place of an image, then you shall enter the Kingdom."**

This call for developing the ability to see the unity in opposites and making harmony from apparent dissonance shows itself in another writer from an even earlier period, Heraclitus the Obscure. He was considered one of the great Greek teachers/philosophers of the pre-Socratic tradition in 500 BC.

Heraclitus said,

> **Equally Nature strives through opposites to bring about Harmony, and not through like things, just as the male unites with the female and not each with one of the same sex. By means of opposites the first union is achieved, and it seems, too, that art in doing this imitates nature. The art of painting consists of mixing the natures of white and black, yellow and red, and producing harmonious pictures with them; and the same with music, by moderating high and low, long and short sounds one harmony is produced. The whole of writing is the combining of consonants and vowels. That which follows is, according to Heraclites the Obscure, the joining together of things, whole and not whole, agreement disagreement, concord and discord, all things are one and from one are all things.**

A Taoist could have written both of the above statements. An appreciation of the paradox that lies in the shifting tides of creation is evident. If we want to live in a way that is healthy, creative, and productive, we only need to learn the art of harmony. Honoring the movement of the unknowable means being willing to embrace all that it offers, both nice and the nasty and making choices. Certainly there are some things we cannot change in our life, the date of our birth, our birth parents, and the culture we find ourselves in are events we cannot alter. We can, however, make choices about the daily actions and thoughts that define our being and move us into the future we are creating. The choices we make say much about our spiritual maturity.

Our awareness of spirit communicates itself through a particular virtue regarding human potential and our connection with our source in nature. When we are engaged in creating harmony, we serve the whole of humanity. This is the reason that the sages always look to nature for their examples.

The view of human body that serves as the foundation of Chinese medicine takes into account the bone, muscle, tissue, and blood of the body as well as the energy that animates them. The focus is on the energy, the binding force. It is the energy or Chi that is seen as the connection between all aspects of life; it is the glue that binds things together. It is through the appreciation of this unifying energy that insight can be gained into the connectivity between one expression of this life energy and another.

This connectedness extends out to include the mental, emotional, and spiritual life of each individual. When we see the human body in this way, the "softening of boundaries" referred to in chapter 2 can be appreciated not as a metaphor, but as a reference to fact. The elements that nourish us are not simply fragments of a separate environment; they are part of the continuum that connects us to all life on the planet.

Life involves the transformation of energy from one state to another. Our ancestors were dependent on being able to read the messages of natural process in order to live. Knowing nature was not a philosophical pastime; it was a survival skill. Watching wind and water, the cycles of growth and decomposition, and the movement of the stars and moon promoted sensitivity to nature that was essential for the planting of crops, the stalking of game, and predicting the seasons. Human life increasingly exists in built spaces where the earth is covered with cement and where vegetation is sparse. As our environment has changed, our senses have been drawn away from nature in its primal state. We only experience it as it is filtered through the mind and hand of man. Our attention is increasingly pulled to the world of human action without the larger frame of reference that lies in natural process. As our experience of nature becomes more abstract, the inherent value of it becomes clouded. We begin to believe that we are separate from the world we live in.

In an essay titled "Good and Bad Reasons for Believing," my favorite scientific enchanter Richard Dawkins makes the following assertion. I should point out that this was originally written for his young daughter and so lacks his usual flair.

> **Lions are built to be good at surviving on the plains of Africa. Crayfish are built to be good at surviving in fresh water, while lobsters are built to be good at surviving in the salt sea. People are animals too, and we are built to be good at surviving in a world full of . . . other people. We "swim" through a "sea of people. Just as a fish needs gills to survive in water, people need brains that make them able to deal with other people."**

If you ever wondered why you have a brain, there's your answer. Lions have the plains of Africa, crayfish have the rivers, lobsters have the ocean, but we simply have each other.

This is a big and beautiful planet that we share with other human beings and millions of creatures very different from ourselves. They all have lessons to teach us, and they are all alive and part of the chain of being. We have been given the ability to both think and feel. Both are valuable gifts, and we should learn to use them both since they are the dual qualities that define us as human. When we separate ourselves off from the connectedness of life, our only option is war with nature. Many scientists and politicians treat the idea of cooperation with nature as a sign of weak sentimentality or lack of trust in the human intellect. They feel that to adapt our actions to suit the health of the planet would be to negate human primacy. This idea allows us to see the importance of all life only in relationship to our own greed, not our own needs. Our basic needs are easily met through application of our innate intelligence.

Our options are simple; our lives depend on our ability to learn nature's laws and respect them. Our authentic self flourishes when we acknowledge and experience our connection with nature. When we lose that connection, we can only value nature in ways that support our own small existence. Nature becomes the "other"—its resources, beauty, or value to the soul become an amusing irrelevance. Living only in the "sea of people" without regard to the fact that our identity is intimately linked to the larger environment isolates us. In this state of separation, our attention is on the current cultural enchantments, and we are blinded to any sense of larger purpose. Because we do not experience it, life requires an intimacy of contact between the source of our being and ourselves. It also requires a realization of that process.

This is how the British philosopher E. F. Schumacher stated it:

> **The extraordinary thing about the modern "life sciences" is that they hardly ever deal with life as such, but devote infinite attention to the study and analysis of the physio-chemical body that is life's carrier.**

In order to bridge the apparent contradiction between the feeling and the thinking self, between the spirit and the matter, requires dynamic concepts based on natural process. These concepts must be capable of describing the world in a way that can be experienced directly and observed without any mediating technology.

We are all taught in school about natural cycles, the way that the atmosphere is cycled through the plant and animal kingdoms in a way that supports life, the way that water is purified, settling through the earth, flowing in rivers, evaporating off the seas, and raining on the land. Images such as these describe the simple elegance of the Gaian body but operate only at the level of the surface. Since the beginning of time, men and women have observed these movements and noticed those same patterns repeated in their own lives. They discovered ways to increase sensitivity to the ebb and flow of energy within and around them and to use it with increased skill. To do this, they experimented with diet and herbs; they developed systems of movement, chanting, and meditation; they discovered ways to heal the sick and clear the mind. All of these skills were aimed at increasing physical, emotional, and spiritual health. Even though the language used to describe these techniques varied depending on environment and culture, they all were focused on the discovery of the authentic self and the ability to live in harmony with nature.

The Organizing Principle

Yin and *yang* are terms that have been passed down through the history of traditional Chinese philosophy from its origins in Taoism. The terms originally referred to the sunny and shady sides of a valley. They are indicators of extremes in any apparent duality. *Yin* and *yang* are not "things"; they are terms that describe the qualities of energy that dominate any phenomena. They are primarily of use in describing the relationship of one thing to another. This means that something may be more yang than something else but can never be yang itself. It is a simple way of classifying phenomena such as states of being, physical structures, or any natural process.

Like many primitive ways of understanding the world, this ancient philosophy was based on thousands of years of observation and experience. It is built on the appreciation that the energy of nature has defined patterns of movement. Living to the fullest can be best achieved and maintained by synchronizing our actions to align with those patterns. To be ignorant of these movements, to ignore them, or to willfully resist them is to swim against the tide. While either endeavor may bring a momentary thrill and challenge, we will eventually be frustrated and swept away.

To navigate the journey of our life, it is helpful to appreciate the rules that govern the strange sea that we find ourselves adrift in. It is important to have tools for navigation and an understanding of the rules of the tides. The primary tool for navigation is our own experience with guidance from the Pole Star of our authentic self and sensitivity to the currents of yin and yang movement.

The stream of energy that creates the world around us as well as the world within us is called Chi. Chi is born out of the interaction of yin and yang and creates the qualities of both the animate and inanimate world. Within the ocean of possibilities, the tides of yin and yang energy create millions upon millions of tiny eddies and currents of energy that interact, producing unique characteristics. The oak tree and the pine have different Chi, anger and sadness have different Chi, sunlight and moonlight all things are created and enlivened by Chi. To restate the ancient Taoist sages, "The One (The Unknowable) creates the Two (Yin and Yang) and the Two creates the Chi and the Three (Yin, Yang, and Chi) create all things." We are capable of perceiving these qualities of Chi through our senses and our feelings. Imagine a set of five strings; each string has a black tab on one end (B) and a white tab on the other (W). On one string, we will write *blue* on the B end and *red* on the W end. On the next string, we will write *passive* on the B end and *active* on the W end; and on the third, we will write *sweet* on the B end and *salty* on the W end. On the next string, *sad* on the B end and *angry* on the W end; and on the last string, we will write *soft* on the B end and *hard* on the W end. Then we will braid these strings with all the black ends and all the white, facing the same direction.

The black end of this braid will have the words *blue, passive, soft, sad*, and *sweet* together; and the white end will have the words *red, active, salty, angry*, and *hard*. Even though there are colors, emotions, tastes, and textures represented, there is a resonance between the terms. They seem to represent a certain tone of experience and feeling; it is the Chi that carries that tone. We associate blue with sadness, soft with passive, and sweet with soft. These associations exist because there is an affinity that unites them. It is the same with the relationship between red and action or anger, or hardening with salty.

These phenomena describe distinct qualities of existence and experience that are easy for us to identify. We use this language of qualities to create a deeper meaning in our communication. It is through the more poetic uses of language that we can speak about the emotional, sensory, and spiritual aspects of our life. The use of metaphor, allegory, and analogy bring life to the stories of Jesus, Buddha, Lao Tzu, and all the great sages of the past. These stories and poems are essential because they indicate a realm of human perception that goes below the surface and into the heart of the vibrational world that unites all things. When we see the world as a living entity and not a "ball of gas or mindless matter," these stories have a great capacity to create a unified vision of life. Seeing life as an integral part of nature lays that framework for the experience of affinity required by the authentic self. Nature is no longer an enemy to be battled—it is our teacher. The Indian guru Anagarika Govinda says it this way:

> **If we look at the world ... with the eyes of the spirit we shall discover that the simplest material object ... is a symbol, a glyph of a higher reality and a deeper relationship of universal and individual forces.**

We are comprised of energy in many forms. The Chi of our ancestors and our environment make up our constitution. We are neither a blank tablet on which our environment etches our destiny or bound to a future dominated by our parents' blood. Our body is nourished daily by the Chi of air, water, food, climate, family, work, sex, and the whole spectrum of interaction with the outside world. Everything in human life has its particular qualities of this life force. Specific qualities of this energy serve to either enhance our affinity with the world or create a barrier for that experience.

States of physical, emotional, and spiritual health are often described as states of balance. This balance is an internal harmonizing of opposites reflected in our ability to create harmony with our environment. The Taoists described living a good life as a process of appreciation and co-operation with the forces of nature. This ancient vision of how the world works is the root of macrobiotic thinking and is fundamental to understanding Oriental medicine. The Taoist philosophy was first written down about 600 BC and certainly reflects much older spoken traditions. Its applications in medicine date back at least four thousand years. An understanding of the terms is helpful for an appreciation of their application in the traditional way of creating a healthy life.

I have used Ohsawa's classifications in regard to food in later chapters since I feel they speak directly to the way we experience food in the body and the relationship of various foods to the environment. This is not classic Oriental medicine as practiced by acupuncturists and herbalists. This distinction is not a concern for everyday use and is only important in the specific treatment of disease using herbs or acupuncture in a prescriptive fashion.

Yin and yang defines qualities of Chi as they are expressed in movement, structure, or function within nature and in human behavior. Here are some basic examples of these qualities.

	YIN	YANG
Movement	Slow	Fast
Temperature	Cold	Hot
Weight	Light	Heavy
Density	Porous	Impermeable
Direction	Peripheral	Central
Biological Life	Vegetal	Animal
Texture	Soft	Hard
Climate	Temperate	Tropical
Season	Winter/Autumn	Summer/Spring

Consider these qualities as the outcome of energy in its contractive phase (Yang) or its expansive phase (Yin). When energy moves toward a point it will produce dense structure, weight, heat and light. When energy expands it creates weightlessness, porous structures, darkness and cold. When we experience a cold (Yin) climate we clasp our arms around ourselves, contract our muscles and move quickly (Yang) to keep warm. In the summer when it is hot (Yang) we want to relax ourselves, we move slowly and want cooling foods (Yin). These activities seem second nature to us because it is natural to seek balance.

Stress is a result of an imbalance of yin and yang. This applies to politics, economics, religion, or the human body. When life is too influenced by a particular extreme, it loses freedom of thought and action. The balanced state is not static; it is a dynamic condition where harmony is achieved between ourselves, the ever changing physical and cultural environment and our personal goals. One of the indicators of health is that we can maintain harmony in our movement toward our goals with the least compromise due to physical, emotional or mental incapacity.

We know and acknowledge states of imbalance in others and ourselves. We may say that someone is "uptight," "cold," or "spaced out" and know exactly what is meant. We even know how to "treat" the problem. We know that the tense person needs to learn to relax, the cold person needs to seek a little warmth and that the spaced out individual needs to focus. In other words—we know that balance is essential. The problem is that there is often no relationship seen between this casual observation and any deeper reality, more importantly we lack the tools to effect a change in the condition. The macrobiotic philosophy encourages us to rediscover this language of the feeling state and the ways it can be used in daily life. The concentration on what we eat and the effect of foods in macrobiotics is important in several regards here.

The wise use of food can help to enhance awareness of natural process. As opposed to other aspects of our environment, food is easiest to control and very direct in its effect. It is possible to experience the Chi of food when we become more conscious of our eating. By becoming more selective to food choices, we can gain a sensitivity regarding the ways that specific foods change our state of well-being. This is an important life skill. Having an intellectual appreciation that certain foods may be more or less detrimental to health is different to being able to literally experience that effect. It is the visceral awareness of how we are affected by what we eat that serves as a practical guide in making healthy choices and contributes to increased sensory acuity.

More primitive approaches to health describe a spiritual and practical view of life as distinct from any specific religious creed. One of those principles is the understanding that while we share much in our humanity, we are all unique creatures. This uniqueness is reflected in our physical, emotional, and spiritual character. Our life purpose is to discover the gifts contained in this character and to express them. We have the ability to make choices in life regarding the sources of energy we draw from to fulfill this potential. We are constantly in the process of creating ourselves through what we take in and how we give our energy back to the world. It is not only mystics who speak of this energy. This is what Agnes de Mille, the famous choreographer, had to say:

> **There is a vitality, a life-force, an energy, a quickening that is translated through you into action, and because there is only one of you in all of time, this expression is unique. If you block it, it will never exist through any medium and will be lost . . . . The world will not have it. It is not your business to determine how good it is, or how valuable, nor how it compares with other expressions . . . . It is your business to keep it yours clearly and directly, to keep the channel open.**

Many of the imbalances in our lives can be seen as a direct result of our lack of understanding of nature and making poor choices. Actions that go against the natural order of nature rebound in harmful effect. This means that lack of harmony in our lives is a metaphor for our thoughts and actions. The thoughts that occupy our minds daily reflect our relationship to Spirit and can manifest clearly as pain or anguish. The disharmonies within that relationship become potential teachings to both individual and society if we accept them as part of the larger drama of life. The threads of connection never stop.

Many people have an aversion to this relationship, they feel that it places "blame" on the sick—this is not true. While some in the alternative health community dismiss the effect of genetics, environment, and the possibility of accidents, I do not. This is not the central issue. We act according to our perception, education, and cultural conditioning. If the actions of our culture create sickness and unhappiness, we must use our power to transform that culture—blame has no place here, neither does the impotence of the "victim." If we are ill, we must educate ourselves and follow the most prudent path to health.

Chapter Seven

Health and Habit

Living in the Comfort Zone

When we extend the discussion of health beyond the realm of physical discomfort to include our whole experience of life, it becomes obvious that establishing health is a transformative process. It entails fundamental changes in both thought and action. It involves a review of the patterns of behavior that have taken away from our true potential.

Health has everything to do with habit. The way we eat, the amount of exercise we get, the ways we think are all habits that can either move us forward to health and happiness or send us down the path to sickness and disappointment. The rituals of daily life can only be adapted for the better if we are clear about our priorities and accept the challenge of acting as if those priorities are important. If we can identify positive goals, we can construct actions that correspond to the achievement of them. It is good to realize that habits are there for a reason. If there were no benefit to us in some way, they would not exist. We talk about our habits as if they attacked us when we were not looking.

There are both healthy and unhealthy habits. We all know people who are or have been addicted to alcohol, cigarettes, overeating, or any number of harmful personal choices. What is curious is that usually the person knows that the habit is harmful. Most habits are not a result of ignorance. I have often asked clients if they could list seven things they could do to improve their health—they all can do it. Not only are we aware of what needs changing but also we have a fairly good idea about what to do about it. If health is about moving forward in life, we can see that the only way a particular action can be considered unhealthy is that it impedes that movement. Some people can have a drink or not have a drink without feeling any pressure one way or the other. Some people can watch TV without feeling the need to do so every night. It is the compulsion that is the problem, the feeling that we are not in control. The issue here is one of freedom.

One question that always arises is if our habits are a choice or governed by our biology. This argument rages on in the scientific community, but a simple review of the literature shows that there is little to indicate anything such as an addictive personality. The influence of genetics in even the most tested arena of alcoholism has been shown to be very slim. Even the genetic factor as a cause in degenerative diseases accounts for only a very small percentage of the cases. That does not mean that there is no relationship; it simply means that the question of habitual behavior and genetics is marginal.

The most common reasons for unproductive habits are physical comfort, a substitution for something else, escape from physical or emotional distress, acting in rebellion, or inflicting self-punishment. These are factors that also play a role in addictive behavior. That's quite a list, but the common denominator is one thing—unhappiness with the life that's being lived. When we are bored or disappointed with our lives, we pursue actions that distract our attention with harmful or even fatal consequences.

Boredom is usually perceived as a lack of interest in what goes on around us, the perception that things are dull, tedious, and repetitious. The state of boredom has been perceived as a normal human trait that can lead to either alienation or action. In modern culture, boredom is a market force. Huge investments are made to distract us from boredom. The act of reflecting on the source of our state of being or doing something creative are replaced by passively viewing the actions of actors or celebrities who personify excitement or the purchase of objects that symbolize success. Only the most jaded would agree that these are healthy options.

Boredom is the exact opposite of healthy vitality. A healthy life is a life of engagement. It is difficult to maintain boredom when our senses are awake, our mind is active, and our body is responsive. Boredom is not a state of rest or relaxation from meaningful action; it is a retreat from it. We must ask ourselves if we really want to become a society of voyeurs, or if there is something more exciting and fulfilling that we could be engaged in. If boredom is the breeding ground for our stagnant rituals of behavior, it makes sense to find the ways that we can enliven the waters.

The habits of health serve to transform, not suppress. They are daily thoughts and actions that bring us into alignment with movement toward that self-actualized state that is our true potential. The steps to moving down that path are not mysterious or complex; they are simple, but not always easy. They always demand attention and a firm sense of purpose.

The process of personal development is not merely transformational but holds within it the seeds of metamorphosis. It is not simply a surface improvement but a deeper shift in form, thought, and function. While each aspect of our life may hold specific challenges, there is a path that lies at a deeper level that requires a more mindful exploration. The tools and techniques that we learn in the process of our own improvement serve all aspects of our life. This path has to do with the substance of the body as well as the nurturing of the mind and spirit. The metamorphosis of the caterpillar to the butterfly is instructive.

The caterpillar grows out of its skin several times; it sheds each constraining casing it has built for one less rigid. When it knows it has exhausted the possibilities of its "caterpillar-ness," it finds a safe place to be and makes a hard shell for the inner work ahead—the complete disassembly of its former self. Within that shell, it dissolves—it turns into caterpillar soup and rearranges itself into something very different. It prepares for a vastly different life. It will no longer crawl from leaf to leaf; now it will fly. But the job of metamorphosis is not finished till the shell of the chrysalis is broken through. The excess tissue of its past life now forms a barrier that must be broken through. It's not an easy job.

It is the work of breaking out of the chrysalis that is essential for the butterfly to have the strength to soar. Once it has breached the shell, it takes a deep breath that pumps body fluids into its damp and crumpled wings, enabling it to take wing. If a well-meaning human were watching the drama of that struggle, they might be tempted to cut the chrysalis and free the butterfly—the butterfly would die. It needs to break out to strengthen its body (and perhaps its butterfly mind). Liberation is always a struggle. It involves digesting the past, the intention to change, and the passionate desire to act. There are no shortcuts. We don't need to worry that we are turning our back on our past. Researchers have shown that the butterfly still remembers the lessons learned in its previous life.

Transformation requires motivation. The hope that things will be better without a desire to change is doomed to fail. The source of this motivating force may come through fear, but fear is easily exhausted. It may come through a spontaneous revelation, but that usually happens to those who have prepared for the event. Most often, the inspiration to change is generated by our imagination and an enlivened mind. It arises when we can clearly see that change is essential—that in fact—our life depends on it. When we reach this exciting conclusion we are willing to take the risks that change entails.

Personal Vision

Our personal vision of who we are in the world is a guiding factor in what we will do. When what we are doing is in alignment with what we really desire, the opportunity for the "flow" experience referred to in chapter 3 moves closer to the surface. This experience—so common among athletes and artists—is available to us all. It is when we are totally engaged in the moment. It is when we are most alive. This state of being is the opposite of boredom; it is the act of total engagement.

The spirit and vision that guides any action has a great influence on the results. Creating health is a profound statement of faith in the process of life. It does not depend on the purchase of a particular product, enrollment in a specific course, or demanding of any special skills. There are simple ways of being that can be realized when we fully desire to manifest them and are willing to change. Of course the first question is, "Change to what?"

In this chapter, I am going to talk about several ideas that are common to many tribal cultures around the world. Some of these ideas have been appropriated in modern culture and used in business or the self-help industry. It is natural that this cultural pollination happens, but often the spirit of the original practice is lost or diluted. The depth of outcome with any technique is relative to the spirit of engagement. The creation of personal vision is one such technique.

Creating a personal vision is not a vision quest. Vision quests are specific tribal rituals that are practiced by Native American tribes from Alaska to South America. They are important rites of passage in the process of moving from child to adult. Adults need a vision to guide them. They most often include preparation and fasting, usually isolation in nature, often specific meditations and serious introspection. Their intent is to establish contact with the higher spiritual guidance for attainment of the authentic self.

This quest echoes shamanic practices in many parts of the world. This spiritual search is similar to the meditations of the knights, ancient kings, and druids of Europe. The search has only one object—to identify and align with our true purpose in life. When we are on the path to our true purpose, the journey of the soul is fully engaged. This highest state of health is one where our daily actions take a larger meaning.

George Ohsawa talked about the pursuit of an infinite dream when describing the macrobiotic ideal of life. Knowing what we are here for and not being swayed from our larger purpose. The scope of this may seem daunting to some, but it is a lesson that can be used according to our desire. It assumes two things. The first is that everyone has a deep sense of purpose in his or her lives, and the second is that we can access that sense of purpose if we don't already know what it is. How we know that purpose is a mystery with many possible answers.

For some, the answer to that mystery lies in the subconscious mind. They say that there is an unfulfilled mission that has called us and that we have buried. I don't know if it makes a difference how it got there, but there it is. When working with clients, I often ask what they would do if they didn't have the responsibilities they have taken on. I often get very inspiring answers, visions that speak to hidden talents and aspirations. They all hold the kernel of something unique that the person has to offer the world. These unfulfilled dreams often go right to the root of the problem. When we are not moving toward the achievement of our dreams, life is drained of purpose.

We all have such dreams and visions that have been put aside, diminished by others, or overwhelmed by circumstance. Those dreams will never go away because they represent our reason for being here. Each dream is unique and seeks expression. The American psychologist James Hillman has compared these seeds of potential as the *diamon* referred to in Greek mythology. The diamon is the guiding spirit of our lives. It is the spiritual companion that is aligned with our higher purpose.

Some people have a strong sense of their diamon at an early age and trust that spirit completely. They will seem destined to pursue their goal from an early age and never waver. Others feel the draw of that spiritual force but are distracted or discouraged from following it. The discouragement usually comes from those who have turned their back on their own vision and are intimidated by anyone who dares to march to a different drum. The social cushion of mediocrity is a powerful weapon against the animated spirit of the seeker.

I have noticed that the idea of following our personal vision is often blown out of practical perspective. Everything that happens in the world bears significance. We need not think that every person must have a personal vision to establish world peace or discover a cure for cancer. We all have an innermost dream of life the way we would like it to be and the way we would like to live it. To some, that dream may be focused on family or community; for some, it may be intellectual or artistic, it may involve building beautiful furniture or playing music. It is internal integrity, not external implications, that is important. When we are moving toward our own integrity, we often discover forks in the road that lead us into places that we did not dream of initially. These lesser-traveled roads may lead us to larger dreams that need attention. It is the movement that is important.

The Land of One Hundred Monkeys

Since the late 1970s, there has been a popular story about how monkeys on an island off the coast of Japan demonstrated a psychic link. The story goes that the monkeys learned a new way of washing their food and that when a critical mass of monkey learned to do this, monkeys on other islands began changing their actions through paranormal communication. Unfortunately the story turned out to be false for those particular monkeys.

There is, however, a tribe of monkeys living on another island that do respond in that way. That island sits on our shoulders, within our heads. Tribes of monkeys that are mischievous, territorial, and often malicious inhabit this island. Their chatter is often referred to as self-talk, but we have to ask, who is talking and who is listening?

When we pass someone talking out loud to themselves on the street, we may think them strange while we are having an internal dialogue about them as we watch. For most people, this internal to-and-fro is a constant flow of opinions. It has a powerful effect on our actions and is often most active when we are faced with a big decision. Whether conscious or unconscious, these internal debates affect what we do and how we feel. Internal conversations can encourage us toward our dreams and goals, or they can freeze us in our tracks. With all these monkeys chattering throughout the day, there are at least two things we can do: the first is to enforce some quiet time and the second is to bring in some better monkeys.

Stress is when the monkeys get really excited. All the cages are rattled. One of the reasons for the extreme reactions to potential stressors is the fact that we have not developed internal skills to create silence. Modern lives are filled with background noise, speech, music, and the electronic hum of the cities. We try to make sense of these sounds and eventually stop hearing out of protection. The inner silence that has been treasured by seekers throughout history is a resting place where the body, mind, and spirit can experience alignment without any other demand. The art of creating this inner silence is usually referred to as meditation—learning to cut off the chatter and experiencing the silence of the soul.

When we concentrate our attention on one point with no expectations and silence our inner voices, we develop a new and peaceful sense of self. When the monkeys are silent and the static is tuned down, the authentic self has the opportunity to gain status in our internal world. The monkeys always rationalize the drama of our lives and fortify the habits that limit us. The quote below is from Carlos Castaneda.

> **We talk to ourselves incessantly about our world. In fact we maintain our world with our internal talk. And whenever we finish talking to ourselves about ourselves and our world, the world is always as it should be. We renew it, we rekindle it with life, and we uphold it with our internal talk. Not only that, but we also choose our paths as we talk to ourselves. Thus we repeat the same choices over and over until the day we die, because we keep on repeating the same internal talk over and over until the day we die. A warrior is aware of this and strives to stop his internal talk.**

One of Castaneda's points here is worth a closer look. We create our external world through our internal dialogue. If our self-talk is dominated by the view that the world is cruel or nasty, we are going to find ourselves in a cruel and nasty world. Whatever we think our life is going to be is probably going to be true. This is convenient because we get to be right almost all the time. It is the negative talk that seems to easily dominate this internal forum. The arguments regarding why we are not smart enough, don't come from the right background, or don't have the right skills undermine our vision and counsel us to accept less.

Our authentic self often only enters the discussion after the event. This happens when we ask ourselves why we didn't speak up, why we didn't respond with more integrity, why we didn't let the light of our own vision shine through. On these occasions, we are not in alignment with our own vision, and the habits of thoughts and actions constructed by the past hold us firmly in place. We are actors in a play with a faulty script that seems designed to make our lives either comic or tragic, but never heroic. There is only one answer to the dilemma—write a new script.

We have written the full story of our life, including the script for the monkeys in the first place. We have certainly had assistance in the preparation, and the plot may reflect events we have experienced or seen, but this is our own masterpiece. It is the story of our past filtered through emotion and a desperate desire to make sense of it all. The story is rationalized by all the powerful enchantments and mythologies of our family, religion, and culture. It is a powerful mix of limited thinking and fear with two interesting factors. Most of the talk is about the past, which we cannot change, and it has all been constructed with little or no conscious effort on our part. It was thrown together with no thought, and yet it runs our life.

The fact that we cannot change the past does not mean we should be governed by it. The fact that many of our ideas about ourselves were constructed without reflection or affinity with our deepest ideals does not mean we need to accept the limitations they represent. We have within us the ability to balance the chatter of our self-talk with messages that resonate with our vision and the values that vision epitomizes. A complement to the inner silence of meditation is the composition of a new description of our life that supports our vision. This means setting clear objectives and supporting them with meaningful actions.

The internal dialogue is usually filled with negation and limitation; significant life goals are often undermined before they have a chance. Self-talk can convince us that our goals are too difficult, too grand, or simply stupid. The creative approach to this is to invent an internal conversation that, at least, balances the chatter if not drowns it out. The use of personal affirmations (see chapter 13) can assist us to move beyond self-set limitations and serve as a springboard for creating a liberated sense of self.

It is unfortunate that this technique has been most closely associated with the development of business, sales skills, and the generation of wealth. Many methods originally developed for introspection, prayer, and personal transformation have become popular as ways to burrow deeper into the enchantment of material success. The self-help industry has largely become a popular proving ground for supposed spiritual development where proof of the divine is established by financial gain. This consumption-driven use of the technique is logical. It shows that when the distinction between "having" and "being" is unclear, everything is for sale. This is where we dress up some of the monkeys in religious costumes so that they become more acceptable.

The mind is not a neutral sponge that absorbs whatever it is exposed to if we are clear in our intention in life and develop awareness. The enchantments of culture depend on an insensitive mind. Consider the fact that the average American is exposed to between one thousand and three thousand advertising messages a day. These messages are designed to feed habits of thought and action. We can train our mind and learn to focus our mental, emotional, and spiritual energy with conscious intent. This is not simply something we can do, this is something that we are designed to do. It is a distressing aspect of our education that the most important life skill—knowing how to operate our mind—is left to chance.

Passionate Intention

The development of a clear vision of our life purpose and the disengagement from social enchantments does not imply a negation of the world as it is. The sea we find ourselves swimming in is filled with equal parts of miraculous and disturbing happenings. The more we allow our authentic self to emerge, the better we become in dealing with the people and events that surround us. With health comes greater judgment regarding what serves our vision and increases the level of integrity in our lives.

The authentic self readily responds to the call of passionate intention. If our vision and our values are important, then they need to be treated with respect. It is important that we know that most monkeys are conservative and communal by nature. The most potent self-talk counsels us not to step out of line, rock the boat, or alienate ourselves from those around us. Most of us do not relish the role of being the eternal outsider; we are communal creatures, and rejection is an unpleasant experience. The challenges to the man or woman who dares to move counter to the enchantments of culture often finds themselves creating friction where none is intended. This friction is not simply internal; it includes those around us.

When we adopt a stance that promotes our personal freedom, we must then extend that freedom to others as well. We are all free to conduct our lives as we see fit. Increased health is not burdened by restrictions but enlivened by informed choice. It is about knowing how things affect our body and mind and making choices that are not driven by compulsion or fanatic zeal. Freedom always requires discipline but discipline is not the goal.

If we choose to avoid a particular food, hold a unique view of life, or devote ourselves to an uncommon cause, it is best done without regret or the need for anyone else to mimic those thoughts or actions. The application of discipline in health needs to be driven by our passionate intention to manifest our vision. We are asked to move beyond the "good or bad" realm of making decisions and instead to ask ourselves if our thoughts and actions serve our vision or do not.

When I was a young boy, we lived in a house with my grandmother. She did all the cooking while my mother was at work. She was a great cook and spent the better part of the day in the kitchen. She loved cooking for the family and anyone who wanted to come. It was her way of expressing her love and care for the family. She only used fresh food, cooked all her own bread and desserts, and every year bottled up pickles and vegetables for the coming months.

In my midtwenties, after eight years of very focused unhealthy living, I changed my diet and started eating according to macrobiotic principles. When the holidays came, I planned out what foods I would take with me to the family feast with certain trepidation. This was the meal that most of the family would look forward to for a month; the menu was always the same, was delicious, and I was messing with it.

When I arrived and moved through the ritual greetings, my grandmother called me aside into the sacred territory of her kitchen. She looked me up and down and said, "I understand that you are on some kind of a diet to be healthy and that you don't eat some of the food that's on the table. Is that right?" I said, "That's right, Gran." She looked at me with a very serious expression and said, "Well, OK, you know what you have to do, but I want you to know one thing. You never got sick eating anything I cooked for you." I was very touched by this thought of hers. I know that she put lots of love in her food, it would be devastating to her to believe her food had made me sick. Aside from that, she was correct, her food was wholesome and always cooked with simple ingredients and care. I told her she was right and that she was the best cook in the world. Her face lit up, and she said, "I love you. Now get out of my kitchen, I've got work to do."

All through dinner, she would wink at me every time I took food from one of her dishes. This was an important lesson to me in several ways, and I am lucky that it happened early in my food adventures. Food is an important bond between families and also friends. Not everyone has such an easy time with the issue of food and family or any other aspect of healthy living. Often the resistance to change can get blown out of proportion and cause serious damage to family ties and friendship. It is important that we are able to respect the right of others to their opinions while we walk the path of our own choosing.

Our personal ethical principles need to stand on their own and be demonstrated in our own life to the best of our ability. The frustrations of conflicting views are best expressed by increased commitment to our own values and a healthy sense of humor. Our actions must speak for themselves. When we communicate our principles through our actions and an openness to engage in dialogue with those who hold other views, we attract more respect for our ideas. Mahatma Gandhi who said, "Be the change you wish to see in the world," best expressed this ideal.

In the following chapters, I am going to take a closer view of some of the main aspects of creating a healthy life that respects our place in nature as well as the development of our true potential. My purpose is to utilize macrobiotic principles and practice and to explore some of the implications of their use.

Natural Body / Natural Mind

Chapter Eight

Food and Culture

The Gift

We are blessed with the warmth and light of the sun, but within the biosphere, there are three sacred gifts that nourish human life—food, water, and air. The contamination of these gifts is a sad commentary on our values. It would be easy to say that the disregard shown for these gifts was a modern phenomena, but it would not be true. For centuries, we have cut down forests to build ships and fouled rivers with disregard for the future. Our ability to turn this tide of ignorance and indifference is a challenge that should excite our most noble and spiritual nature. This transformation will require vast resources and political will, but must be translated into daily action on the part of those who value life. My focus on the issue of food is only one part of the puzzle, but it is an important one.

There is no single issue that illustrates how our cultural enchantments pull us away from a healthy relationship with the planet than our attitudes regarding what we eat. It is on the inner surface of the respiratory tract and in the intestinal mucosa where the apparent distinction between the outer and the inner disappear. It is here where the energy of the environment is received for the miraculous transformation of life. The prayers of thanks that our ancestors gave before eating speaks to the knowledge that food bestows the gift of life. It is such a simple fact—without food, we die.

When a small portion of the planetary population, those living in the wealthy countries, undermines their health through overconsumption of food while malnutrition and starvation are epidemic among the poor, we know that the sacred qualities of food are being ignored. The relationship between these extremes of nutritional exploitation should not surprise us.

The ecological and economic impact of the modern diet lead us back again to the inescapable fact of our unity with Gaia. When we disrupt that relationship, the effects of that disruption ripple out to effect society and nature. Upsetting the balance of that relationship is catastrophic. This is not the punishment of an angry god; it is simple cause and effect—it is natural justice.

If statements regarding the Gaian principle of unity are correct, it means that the diet that produces optimum physical health should also be one that produces economic justice, promotes a more peaceful society and environmental stability. It is easy to dismiss the possibility of this idea as being utopian, but it is true. It is also true that it is possible to remedy this imbalance. Our capacity to make productive and healthy changes to the growing, manufacturing, and production of food will revolve around our ability to clearly see the ways that our cultural enchantments have perverted that relationship.

Waiting for big government, big health care, big science, or any social institution to come to the rescue is time wasted. Large institutions are like the *Titanic*: the problem is not that the impending disaster goes unnoticed; the problem is that the ship is too big to turn quickly. The issue of healthy food is too important to be given over to a bloated bureaucracy. Science, medicine, and business have all contributed to the drift away from a healthy diet. Each in their own way has created confusion and distraction from the central issues.

Food and Science

We need to consume food that is productive of health and vitality. As we will see, this is not a difficult task. Even with the challenges of living in an environment where we are exposed to poor air and water quality, healthy dietary needs are easily met in the Western world. The requirements for protein, fats and carbohydrates, vitamins and minerals have not changed much over the centuries. Given this simple fact, we will have to ask ourselves why then there is so much uncertainty about what to eat.

Much of the confusion has to do with the misapplication of science and the resulting lack of common sense that goes with it. Contrary to the mythology that all science is unbiased, science is for sale. This is particularly true with regard to nutrition. The bulk of the research being done in nutrition has to do with the specific role of micronutrients, not food. This is an important distinction since it is based on the false premise that there is something deficient with food in its natural form or that finding out the biological function of specific nutrients will somehow resolve the diet-disease connection. Neither of these premises is true.

The science of nutrition was developed primarily to discover the cause of specific nutritional deficiencies. It did a good job. We realized that vitamin C deficiency caused scurvy and that calcium deficiency created bone loss. It is good to know these things, but how do we use the information? Do we conclude that since vitamin C prevents scurvy, we should take it in capsule form just in case? Or that since milk has plenty of calcium we need to drink it to prevent bone loss? These popular urban mythologies were driven not by science but by industry. The orange growers loved the vitamin C discovery, and the dairy farmers were ecstatic about calcium; it was an advertising bonanza. The fears of nutritional deficiency continue to drive the science of nutrition beyond any sensible borders. It has become the official handmaiden of the food industry. Every time the function of a new micronutrient is confirmed and labeled, it is identified as the missing link to health and happiness or the cure to what ails you.

A major problem is that it is next to impossible to study human nutrition with any scientific precision. You would have to lock large populations into laboratories and feed them specific nutrients; you would have to dissect them and study their guts. We can be sure that the volunteer lists would fall short of the numbers essential for a valid study.

Humans eat a diverse diet and have different constitutions; they have vastly different activity levels and live in different environments. All of these factors confound true scientific investigation of what people eat and how it affects them. It steers the primary function of nutritional science to the study of specific nutrients removed from the foods they exist in and devoid of any relationship to their function in a person's diet or specific environmental influence. In other words, it has very little to do with what people eat. There is one area of nutritional research where this is not the case. That is the study of nutritional epidemiology.

Epidemiology is the study of the causes of disease in large populations. If the sample population is large enough and diverse enough, the big picture becomes very clear in terms of the effects of diet. It is these studies that surface with regularity, create dramatic headlines, cause concern, and then fade away like a bad dream. The studies consistently show the same thing—the modern diet is killing us. This is the only "fact" we should be focused on, but we are easily swayed by considerations of another kind. There are simple reasons why our attention is deflected from the fact that eating fast food, junk food, and chemical brews filled with bubbles and sugar is causing disease. The reasons that these facts do not translate into what we eat have to do with the manipulation of science in the service of business and culture.

It is the bad science that fuels our collective amnesia. This feeds the cowardice of government and many scientific institutions when faced by the monstrous power of business interests. When bad news about diet is presented in the media, the first response is usually from a government health spokesperson assuring us that the study is being reviewed and that no one should panic. The most common advice given is that people should moderate their consumption of the toxic waste being sold and be "reasonable" till told otherwise. "A little bit wouldn't do you any harm. After all, you're still breathing." Everyone knows that the government study will be inconclusive and that the industry providing the offending products will trot out their nutritional experts to point out the "flaws" in the study. These experts will seldom be called to task to prove the exact flaws being referred to or to address the studies in a public forum. The purpose of this puppet show is to slow the flow of information down so that people forget there was a problem in the first place.

The food industry has legions of scientific advisors and employees whose primary function is to legitimize their products. The fact that you can prove almost anything contains beneficial ingredients for health makes it easy to deflect criticism even if the beneficial nutrient is one available from hundreds of less harmful sources. The use of science for the purpose of marketing poor-quality foods and to rationalize the use of harmful chemicals used in food production creates confusion and stifles change. This confusion paralyzes most people. If the scientists can't agree, then making any change could be useless. This is especially true when we are presented with such a wide spectrum of options that require no change at all.

The enchantment with scientific advancement feeds our hopes and dreams. Weekly we are presented with uplifting promises of scientific breakthroughs that grant permission to be reckless. If a newly discovered micronutrient seems to benefit people with heart disease, why cut down the fat? If a new gene is found that predicates some folks to being obese, why bother with exercise? If eating one particular food can protect you from cancer, you would be silly to not just add it in along with the hamburger. One of the fundamental enchantments of nutrition and medicine is the search for the single secret cause. The promise is that some new discovery will be made that allows us to behave any way we want without being harmed. Till that bright and shiny day, we will just have to have faith.

Health and Medicine

Quite logically when people have questions regarding health, they refer to medical opinion. The assumption is that if a person is qualified to diagnose disease, prescribe medication, and perhaps to perform surgery, they certainly must know a lot about health. Unfortunately this is seldom the case.

The medical systems in most countries are specifically designed to treat disease once it has presented itself through symptoms or has been discovered through screening. The prevention of disease and the skills of healthy living are not on the agenda. Of course there are individuals who rise above this assertion, but they are rare. Simply put, helping people get healthy is not the job that physicians are trained for. Physicians are trained to treat the sick. The amount of time spent on topics like nutrition in medical school is next to nothing. The training that most doctors receive is aimed toward diagnosis and treatment because that is what they are going to be doing. When they are in practice, a good deal of study time will be spent just keeping up with prescriptive guidelines for new pharmaceuticals being released and understanding new technical procedures. They have their hands full with damage control. It's a big job.

We tend to view doctors as heroes in our culture. Look at how many popular television programs have hospital settings. Doctors have control over life and death; they can discover hidden symptoms and dispense the healing sacrament of medication. There is no doubt in my mind that they do difficult and often thankless work; unfortunately they don't know much about how to keep you out of the hospital in the first place.

I have had many people respond to lectures about a healthy diet say, "If this is right, why doesn't my doctor know about it?" Even better is when people are ill and changing their diet for the better have their doctor tell them that it might be dangerous for them to change. There is seldom a reason put forward; a doctor doesn't need to have one. When in a bind, doctors will refer to nutritionists for an explanation. I must remind you here that nutritionists are the people who design hospital food. I rest my case on that reason alone.

Many years ago a close family member was in admitted to a hospital in London with a in a coma. When she recovered I started to bring in healthy meals for her and was forced to run the gauntlet of the nutritionists since she was in a "diet restricted unit." Every item needed an explanation and justification. I was reluctantly told the food was approved but each meal had to pass inspection. After the meals were cleared away the doors to the unit were pushed open by a sprightly woman pushing a cart filled with candy and soft drinks that the patients could buy. The profits were donated to a worthy medical cause. When I pointed this surreal fact out to the nutritionist at my next food inspection she simply shrugged and said, "Well everyone likes a little candy." How right she was. The inaction of the medical community in the field of disease prevention is a sad commentary on priorities. We know what causes the most deaths. In a publication by the American Department of Health and Human Services in 1993, it was reported that

> **two-thirds of premature deaths are caused by poor nutrition, physical inactivity and tobacco. That death rate is 5 times more than the number of people killed by guns, HIV, and drug use combined.**

Poor nutrition, exercise, and habitual smoking are things that can be handled simply. Preventing two-thirds of all premature deaths would be a very impressive goal, but we have decided to go down another path. The most common treatments for major or minor health problems are pharmaceuticals.

For pharmaceutical companies, sickness is big business. You don't have to be a conspiracy theorist to know that. Billions of dollars each year are made by this industry. To a pharmaceutical firm, health is actually bad for business. New illnesses are identified every year that require new medications. In some cases, these newfound illnesses are located and labeled with the assistance of the very companies who just happen to have a cure in hand. The greatest areas of growth in this industry lies in treatment for diseases that could be prevented and/or emotional disorders that are continually redefined to include almost everyone who is having a bad day. If this aspect of health care is not addressed, we are not having an honest conversation.

There is no question that we have become a drug-dependent culture. The turning to drugs for every health problem creates a mind-set that is just as common in the hospital as it is on the mean streets of any urban area. It is estimated that about ten thousand people die in America each year from the effects of illegal drugs. This is an issue that draws media attention on a regular basis and has resulted in billions of dollars of public money spent on the "War on Drugs." Every political party has a drug policy to combat this threat to our culture. Unfortunately we are not giving the same concern for the one hundred thousand hospitalized patients who, according to the *Journal of the American Medical Association*, die yearly from properly prescribed drugs. This figure is amazing especially when we add in the more than two million who suffer from serious side effects. The people taking the street drugs are well aware of the dangers; people taking a prescription are not.

In a 1995 report by Dr. Richard Besser of the Centers for Disease Control and Prevention, it stated that iatrogenic (doctor-caused) death in America had reached epidemic proportion. According to Dr. Besser,

> **A definitive review and close reading of medical peer-review journals and government health statistics shows that American medicine frequently causes more harm than good. The number of people having in-hospital adverse drug reactions to prescribed medicine is 2.2 million.**

In the same report, it was noted that the number of unnecessary antibiotics prescribed annually for viral infections was twenty million. When medical mistakes are one of the main causes for death, we need to be worried—very worried.

The problem does not lie with medicine alone. A drug is a quick and easy way to handle overloaded medical systems. The general population demands the very best treatment. As long as the drug solution is put forward as the only effective treatment and prevention is given little attention, then that is where the demand will be. I remember having a conversation with a young doctor friend of mine in London who tried to get his patients to understand the need for good nutrition and to take them off drugs that were not really helping them. He was abused and reported for malpractice. His patients wouldn't budge. The only way things could change is that as much attention and expense were devoted to education, as is to useless or dangerous treatment.

The logical extension of the drug philosophy is the nutritional supplement industry. Taking a pill to fix things is part of our culture. With little or no understanding of the power of food, a population filled with the fear of disease is led to believe that taking specific nutrients in the form of a pill or powder can fill the gap and avert dietary imbalance. This is a sad situation since the basic intuition is correct—the food is deficient; it is the answer that is off center. If broccoli and carrots are helpful in the prevention of cancer, why not take ten pounds of them reduced down to a capsule? While supplements may be needed in some situations, the widespread belief that they will make up for a bad diet is delusional.

Food, Business, and the Environment

The next reason we don't make changes in our diet is that we don't want to give anything up. The distinctly American dream of having it all is rapidly permeating affluent societies all over the world. This is perhaps more true with food than any other sector of the consumer market. Food is big business—huge business. Food companies do over $800 billion a year in business, and the industry is increasingly concentrated into a handful of transnational corporations.

Only five companies control 90 percent of the global grain supply. Eighty-one percent of all American beef is in the hands of four processors. The world tea market is governed by three corporations; and the United Nations estimated that Wal-Mart, the dominant force in the global grocery trade, has profits larger than three-quarters of the world's countries. All of these companies operate according to their own rules. The political influence that the food industry has speaks to the central position it has in the national economy of Western nations. The true symbol of financial vigor the world over is the appearance of hamburger and fried chicken franchises. We are led to believe that we can have our cake and eat it too—and we do love our cake.

One of the key benefits of affluence is abundant food. Going hungry is the ultimate sign of failure in wealthy societies unless it is in the service of spiritual enlightenment or gaining the size 0 body of a fashion model. If we have a meager budget, we want lots of food, especially food that excites our taste buds and fills our bellies. If we have lots of money, we want exotic foods, imported from great distances with sophisticated and subtle tastes. It is no coincidence that the poor are subjected to the unhealthiest foods in the American and Western European diet. The fast-food purveyors of high-fat, high-sugar, high-protein foods with low nutritional content are focused on the young and the poor. The large portions and low cost are seductive. The true cost of their diet will be carried by the burden of rising rates of diabetes, heart disease, and cancer. Obesity, once the exclusive domain of the wealthy, is now available on a budget. Anyone can afford the double cheeseburger with fries.

It is worth noting that much of the marketing of fast foods appeals directly to the young and also to a generation that refuses to acknowledge the ageing process. The teenagers of the 1950s and 1960s were the first group of teens who were a real market force. It was a generation raised on burgers and shakes. Old habits die hard.

When I was in my teens, those fast foods were considered "kids' food." The drive-in restaurants and soda shops were filled with teens and families only went for a "treat for the kids" you seldom saw adults eating there. This was a diet that was not reflected in family or inherited culture; it was a diet invented by business. It was sculpted to fit the image of speed, easy consumption and a kind of casual disregard for food. It was the food of the future, it was science fiction food. The postwar diet of "convenience foods" was sold as a way to escape the drudgery of the kitchen. It was food that was supposed to be clean, nutritious, and cheap; but the small print didn't talk about the ill health and environmental cost of this exciting new enterprise.

On the opposite end of the spectrum from the fast foods is the rise in exotic food consumption among the wealthy and near wealthy. Speciality food shops and natural food stores are quickly becoming high-ticket delicatessens for the educated and high end of the market. Driven by increased environmental and health concerns, these stores have been steadily driven by consumer demand into the conventional supermarket grove to become food extensive food boutiques. To expand market share, there are an increasing number of products that are better "organic" versions of the snack-food, fast-food culture but still bear many of the social costs associated with that approach to eating.

This phenomenon is problematic in that the general quality of the foods is usually healthier, often organically grown, and tends to support regional agriculture. It has also broadened the appeal of good quality foods but the important issue is that the movement to a healthy diet must exist within the larger reality of social justice and environmental stability. This will mean that consumers must be willing to make larger changes in what they eat other than switching over to tofu cheesecake and organic cheese from a small village in the Swiss Alps. Invariably it means that more people need to learn to cook simple food from basic ingredients.

The food business has effects on world health, economy, and the environment that are unrivaled. The transnational corporations that control the growing, manufacture, packaging, and distribution of food have an annual turnover larger than many countries. War or peace, poor or rich, everyone requires food to live. These companies are not in business to deliver healthy food to your local market; they are in business to make the most money possible. They do this regardless of the implications of their business on human life or the environment unless forced to do so by consumer pressure or government regulation. The exceptions to this are few when compared to the size of the industry, and they are to be applauded and supported. They are not the major players.

For the most part, the food industry is operating exactly as would be expected. As Frances Moore Lappe said in 1989,

> **The market left to its own devices will concentrate wealth and purchasing power and therefore undermine its usefulness in meeting human needs. But a government responsible to majority interests can make rules and allocate resources to counteract the tendency toward concentration. These two instruments of economic life need not be in competition.**

The food industry has produced its profit by producing cheap food for the wealthy nations on the back of environmental destruction and the exploitation of cheap labor. It does all this without much scrutiny and often with government subsidy and tax relief. The peculiar fact is that much of the subsidy goes to supporting sectors of the food industry that are most questionable in health terms. Sugar production, cattle ranching, and dairy farming have all prospered with tax breaks and subsidy while the uses of their products are consistently called to question. This cozy relationship is dramatically exposed in government nutritional reports that advise consumers to "cut down on saturated fats" rather than to reduce meat and milk.

Recently, over three hundred oncologists in America signed a petition by the Cancer Project calling for the federal government to review nutrition policy. Among their requests was a review of the over $70 billion in American food subsidies of which three-quarters went to producers of sugar, oil, dairy, meat, and alcohol. This was compared with less than 1 percent that was given to fruit and vegetable farmers. Corn is one crop that is subsidized and is mostly used as cattle feed and to make high-fructose corn syrup (it sounds healthier than sugar, doesn't it?). The price of this ingredient in food manufacturing has gone down by 30 percent in the past thirty years while the cost of vegetables has risen by 50 percent. It is because of these subsidies that in many restaurants a hamburger costs less than a salad. It is the ultimate irony that some of the excess created by these subsidies are then distributed to schools and institutions, assuring that schools suffering from ever-decreasing funds rely on government meat and dairy while the parents lobby for healthier meals in those very schools.

We are regularly told that there is not enough food to feed the growing population of the planet. While it is true that population is a problem, there is plenty of food to feed everyone—not later—right now. The issue is what we do with what we grow. The worldwide production of food is focused on growing grain and beans. This is a good idea. The problem is that we feed most of it to animals, and that's a bad idea unless you are in the animal business.

Huge tracts of land are cleared yearly to grow food for animals. To claim that this is essential to feed the world is a simple lie. The cost to world environment is unimaginable. The same politicians who wring their hands about global warming are not interested in curtailing the one industry that creates the greatest havoc. The deforestation of the Amazon basin alone produces a net loss of valuable forestlands that are essential to offset the carbon-hungry needs of the industrialized and developing world. Besides the denuding of the forests, indigenous people are driven off their land, and small farmers are pushed off to the side. The economy of this exercise is fascinating.

In the last forty years, we have leveled almost half of the rain forests in the world so that we can give them pasture. (There goes renewed air to breathe.) In America, we give the cows fifty-six million acres of land for hay production for livestock and only set aside four million for vegetables for human consumption. (There goes the soil.) But our four-legged friends need to drink as well as eat. It takes twelve thousand liters of water to produce one four ounce beef patty. (Oops, there goes the water.) Talk about love—is there anything we wouldn't do for these cows. It would be instructive for everyone in North America and Europe to adopt a cow, except they don't make good houseguests.

You can just imagine with all that eating and chewing of cuds there must be a downside. The U.S. Environmental Protection Agency estimates that livestock waste has polluted more than twenty-seven thousand miles of rivers. This is starting to look pretty bad but there is more. Cows belch and pass wind creating over 2,622 kilos of methane every year each. That means that if you were to drive a Land Cruiser or any of those vehicles that are designed for the invasion of a small country, you would be producing only 30 percent less methane than if you owned your own gassy cow.

In these days of enlightened capitalism and free markets, it is unfashionable to suggest that governments exercise their power to protect the citizenry from the dangers of unregulated business, but that is just what needs to happen. That, combined with an unseemly surge of common sense from consumers, could dramatically improve the health of the world population as well as that of the planet. These changes would not take decades to create positive results. The changes required are simple to do but difficult to achieve unless priorities are clearly defined. The top priority must be healthy food that has not been contaminated by chemicals in its growth or processing or been produced at the expense of the world's poor.

Let Them Eat Junk

Human society has been putting additives in food since the beginning of history. We have used salt, herbs, spices, and a wide variety of methods to flavor, preserve, and enhance what we eat. There have also been those who would add chalk to flour or paint the grey meat red. The problem lies when the field of food chemistry becomes so sophisticated that even a fairly prudent consumer is fooled. If presented with most of the foods in the supermarket without artificial coloring, emulsifying, flavoring, and preserving, we would be repulsed.

Large studies like the China-Oxford-Cornell Diet and Health Project have proven once again what every sensible study of nutrition has shown before it. A diet that is based on complex carbohydrates and plant-based protein with an adequate variety of fruits and vegetables shows a marked decrease in the types of disease we suffer in North America and Europe. Such a diet also helps most people find their healthy weight if they are getting even moderate exercise. The problem is that there is little profit in these foods.

Many people pride themselves on the fact that they eat junk food. There is an increasingly prevalent attitude that consuming junk food and other foods, which are detrimental to health, is in some way endearing or a defiant stand against being told what to do. The value of food has been so obscured that cynicism reigns, and anyone who attempts to eat in a way that is counter to the national habit is peculiar or even anti-social.

It is certain that the way we eat is one of the most important aspects of healthy living. It is also true that to really change our diet significantly will challenge many contemporary myths of being. America's contribution to world cuisine is the snack. This is food that is often devoid of nutrition, filled with chemical enhancers, created to produce nothing but money and a bloated stomach. The fact that these foods are targeted toward the children of the world is a very sad commentary on our cultural values. The advertising for many of these products promotes their consumption as much as an act of social belonging as it does because they are tasty. Snack foods, fast foods, chips and dips, colas, and candies are quickly becoming the sustenance of America and spread to wherever there is a desire to replicate the perceived cache of American style. The modern swing toward a diet high in fat, low in fiber, high in protein, low in vegetables, and laced with sugar and chemicals will kill you. Diets high in fat are linked to increased risk of several cancers, most notably breast, colon, prostate, and perhaps pancreas and ovaries. It doesn't even seem to matter whether the type of fat is saturated or monosaturated; the results are similar. The sources of these fats in America are meat, dairy products, cooking fats, and salad oils. A similar dietary profile is connected to heart disease and diabetes, namely high fat, sugars (sometimes in the form of alcohol), and low fiber. The way that this risk is communicated to the public is further evidence of the smoke and mirrors of enchantment. The most stated critique of the high-fat, high-protein, sugar-laden diet that has become the modern standard is that it causes obesity. This is like saying that cigarettes should be avoided because they make you cough! You seldom, if ever, hear it said that the diet will kill you—it's the obesity that's the problem. Are you weeping yet?

Our Daily Bread

The domination of poor-quality food in affluent countries is largely a function of "added value." Each time a raw ingredient is processed, there is more money to be made. If rice can be hulled, polished, and then partially cooked, have nutrients added to replace some of those that have been wasted, profit can be garnered at each stage of the operation. The "added value" here is, of course, laughable since the final product is inferior to when it started. The same can be said of the overuse of animals in the food chain, the animals "add value" as well as the processing of the meat or dairy foods into a wide variety of products that started out as raw milk or a cow in a field. There is no place where the impact of the food industry produces the most harm to human and planetary health than in the growth and processing of grain and beans.

When governments all over the world produce dietary guidelines, the graphic model that is invariably used is the food pyramid. The food pyramid shows what foods should be used for optimum nutrition in a clever graphic that places the most important foods at the base and other foods in diminishing quantities as the pyramid becomes smaller at the top. It is a simple and quite helpful graphic with two exceptions. The first exception is that, in America, it could not be further from reality and second that the issue of quality as opposed to quantity is totally ignored.

The base of every food pyramid I have seen, the foods that provide the foundation for a healthy diet, are the cereal grains. This goes for the American ideal to the Asian and the Mediterranean model. Cereal grains and beans have been the bedrock of the human diet since the agricultural revolution thousands of years ago. Coupled with beans, the cereal grains provide the widest range of vegetable-based nutrition on the planet. This is a well-known fact with the exception of the occasional fad diet that decries carbohydrates without distinguishing the issue of refined and unrefined varieties. This has led the population to believe that eating white bread, pasta, and commercial varieties of "brown" bread are natural staples of a healthy diet.

The difference between refined and unrefined grain is an important issue. It is simply the fear of making changes in the economy that prohibits the message to be put forward with the same vigor that the antismoking campaign was pursued. I will revisit this issue in terms of the health benefits of making a shift from refined grains to whole grains in later chapters. Cereal grains have an important place in agricultural societies reflected in their mythology. In North and South America, corn was represented by goddess figures such as the Corn Mother or the Mayan belief that human beings were made of corn. Many Asian tribes pay respect to special rice deities, and in Laos, there is a belief that there is a special quality of energy that is only shared by humans and rice. The Greek goddess of the grains was Demeter who blessed life with the harvest. These stories are a reflection of our ancestors' respect for the central place taken by cereal grains in human society. Even the Lord's Prayer includes the line "Give us this day our daily bread."

The shift to whole foods from refined foods is no longer the message from the fringe but the conclusion of leading health professionals. The empty appeals for moderation are something like counseling an addict to just use a little less heroin in their next fix. When we allow soft drink purveyors to "sponsor" schools that agree to use only their beverage or award grade school achievements with free pizzas, we must ask where our common sense has gone. We must also ask why we have become deadened to the profound effects that eating in such a damaging way produces. Could it be that, like the addict, we have crossed the line where what was once a pleasurable experience has now taken control over our lives?

The dilemma we face involves learning a new way to nourish ourselves that lies outside the manipulation of business and the confusion of nutritional science. It is a challenging task since the messages are buried deep in our culture and are constantly fortified and fueled by the fear of sickness. Part of the process involves becoming skilled at knowing how our bodies respond to the environment we live in and to become sensitive to the effects that foods have on our vitality, sensitivity, and behavior. It is not simply the physical degeneration that is worrying but the effect that our present patterns of eating have on our overall behavior that should give us cause for concern. Since the body is one fully integrated community of cells, the effects of physical imbalance can be traced outward to include the effects of this imbalance on the mind, the emotions, and our personal sense of being.

Part of the solution to this dilemma has to do with rediscovering how the energy of creation—the lessons of wind and water—can be applied to our daily patterns of living. We have a great storehouse of knowledge available to us. The most valuable resource of this wisdom lies in the understanding of indigenous peoples throughout history. This knowledge often requires a translation to meet modern needs but still holds the practical value of common sense, practicality, and effectiveness. Most importantly, it is a way of empowering our own ability to care for ourselves in a way that supports the very best qualities of our humanity.

Chapter Nine

Food and Health

The Price of Convenience

Aside from the ability to breathe, it is what takes place in our digestive tract that most governs our physical health. The intestinal system is a vital environment consisting of consumed foods, enzymes, and digestive juices manufactured by the body as well as extensive colonies of microorganisms usually referred to as the intestinal flora. The intestinal environment is contained within the body, but "it is not us yet." The function of digestion is to break down the food so that it can be absorbed and utilized by the body. Over five hundred bacterial species live in the human intestinal tract; most synthesize vitamins, ferment carbohydrates, convert lactose and other sugars. They also inhibit the growth of pathogenic bacteria (those that cause sickness). To have an image of the complexity of this environment, the human body is comprised of about ten trillion cells, and ten times that number of microorganisms inhabit the human gut. Either what we eat on a daily basis supports the ecology of the internal soil we grow out of or it doesn't.

Our ability to maintain health is dependent on the vitality of this internal world. Macrobiotics and many other natural approaches to a healthy diet aim to restore and enliven this inner world. The fact that we can consume foods that are destructive to this process and still live is often seen as an enticement for abuse rather than a testament to the beauty of human design.

Human beings are complex organisms. That complexity goes beyond the physical complexity of our brain and nervous system; it extends out into our cultural, environmental, and spiritual lives. We roam all over the world and are not confined to a specific environmental niche; we form groupings with vastly different ways of seeing the world and interacting with it. To pretend that any particular diet will suit everyone is a fallacy.

One of the most common problems in explaining the macrobiotic approach to health is that there is no such thing as the macrobiotic diet; there is simply a way of understanding food and the ways that food affects us. In a later chapter, I will discuss a sensible way of integrating this approach to eating in daily life, but first it is essential to reflect on some of the factors that influence this way of eating. Some of these considerations are directly related to physical health, some are ethical influences, and some speak directly to creating a greater energetic balance between the environment and ourselves. The purpose is to create an enhanced experience of what it is to be alive.

When we try to double-guess nature, we always fail. The reason we fail is because the natural food chain is already perfect—any tinkering can only degrade it. Nutritional science seems to be obsessed with creating a perfect diet, but for whom is that diet for? Is it for an eighty-year-old woman who weighs only 125 pounds and lives in Miami, Florida, or that twenty-eight-year-old, two-hundred-pound carpenter in Oslo, Norway? Does environment make a difference; does activity, does body type? Of course they do. Without a vision that embraces the dynamics of life as it is lived, we are placing our faith in what happens in a test tube. Without a compass, we cannot find true North.

Eating has always been seen as a sacred act. It is the process of taking in the energy of life in its most tangible form. It represents the transformation of life energy from air, sunlight, water, and soil. It nourishes not only the body but also the mind and the soul. As our culture becomes increasingly divorced from the growing of food and the alchemy of cooking, we lose our way and entrust food selection and production to industry. Under the slogan of convenience, we hand over this most important of daily actions to commercial enterprise. It is a bargain that turns out to have a horrific cost to both our mind and our body.

If the price we pay for the modern diet is physical disease the effects on our minds is equally, if not more, disturbing. Study after study has shown that eating a diet that is calorie rich and nutrient poor has a huge impact on the mental development of the young. When you combine this information with research showing the highly suspect effect of food additives, you could start to wonder why it is exactly these foods do not come with a health warning. Studies such as that conducted by Dr. Bernard Rimland in California showed that by giving nutritional supplements to hyperactive children, the results were better than drug treatment. In a 1991 article in *Psychopathology*, Dr. Poldinger from the Basel University compared antidepressants and a specific nutrient and showed greater improvements in depression, anxiety, and insomnia with no side effects. This does not mean that every physical or mental disorder can be cured by diet or that nutritional supplements should replace a good diet. It indicates that for many, the answer to their distress lies in what they eat daily.

Unfit for Human Consumption

One of the reasons our modern diet produces imbalances in our health and behavior is because we have radically changed the pattern of eating in recent years through ignorance of its importance. Since we have the capacity to ship foods long distance and preserve them chemically or through refrigeration, we have created dietary chaos. Our contemporary diet is comprised of foods that have been fragmented, overprocessed, and artificially "enhanced" for economic reasons and without thought to the repercussions.

Much of what is eaten in modern society is simply unfit for human consumption. The thousands of man-made substances now used to color, flavor, emulsify, and preserve our food are alien to our biological history. The motivation for their use is purely economic. Our bodies quite simply do not know how to use them. There is still a strong tendency to view the body as a machine without fully acknowledging the subtleties of human sensitivity. It is felt by many conventional nutritionists that as long as there is enough of the basic constituent nutrient in the diet, that health, or at least the lack of dramatic symptoms, can be maintained. Little attention is paid to the importance of the quality of these nutrients and the manner in which they are consumed.

Our body has evolved over millions of years and has an organic familiarity with foods taken in their natural form. Most foods, in their natural state, contain a fine balance of nutrients that maximize the nutritional impact of the food. Many foods contain buffering agents that actually help redress excess in a particular nutrient. It is impossible for nutritional science to improve on foods in their natural state. Outside of the traditional methods of cooking, pickling, and fermenting, modern food science has done nothing to improve the quality of one single food. All the manipulation done to our basic foods has been in the service of the marketplace, not the health of society.

The appeal of the so-called convenience foods is "apparent flavor," ease of purchase and use, and low price—all are illusions. The issue of flavor is a lovely example of physical manipulation. Three flavors that excite the taste buds more than any are fat, salt, and simple sugar. There is speculation that this is true since they were rare in primitive diets. These are the three dominant flavors in junk food. The actual substance of the food is irrelevant, the surface taste could be added to cardboard, and the result would be the same. An oily, salty chip made of any mashed vegetable or animal substance tastes appealing to senses that have been desensitized by poor-quality food. The same is true with sugar. When we add in the chemical flavoring agents that convince us that there is a strawberry in there somewhere even though it's not on the ingredients list, we are helpless. I once picked up a frozen dessert in a British supermarket (where most of my research takes place) and found out that despite the product being called a strawberry cream cake, there were no strawberries and no cream in it. After the water, sugar, and nondairy stuff, there was a long list of chemicals as ingredients. It was a diet product. The food industry counts on you losing your sense of taste as well as your good sense in order to keep turning out the junk.

"Food science" can now give petroleum jelly the texture, taste, and smell of apricot jam and make almost anything taste like chicken. Vegetarians need not despair. The increased number of people who wish to avoid meat provide a growing marketing opportunity. Soy protein and other vegetable-based fibers can be woven to replicate most meat textures and flavored to meet the need. You can have a soy hot-dog if you lace it with enough fats, salt or spices and pretend it's the real thing.

The convenience aspect of prepackaged foods is an interesting one that begs the question, "How much time a day is your health worth?" The family table used to be a regular feature till the mid-1950s. I remember distinctly the introduction to our home of the first TV dinners. You could pop the aluminum tray in the oven, go about your business for half an hour, and then remove the foil top and have the meat and two veg. The whole idea was that you could watch TV and eat them; my father even went out and bought four spindly trays with fold-out legs to put the TV dinners on. They were terrible, but they were really convenient. No one in our small family liked them, and we moved back to the table in short order. We had to deal with the inconvenient problem of cooking.

The most dramatic changes in food quality have occurred since the end of World War II. The modern food industry owes much to the food technology invented during the war. To produce edible foods that could be shipped thousands of miles and last for months in containers, food chemistry was called to the forefront. At the end of the war, this technology was transformed into the rage for convenience foods. These were the foods that were going to free the women of the world from the burden of the kitchen. What they really produced were foods that have ruined our health and created a culture of consumer dependence on the food industry. Food that has been grown is disappearing and being replaced by food that has been manufactured. The biological integrity established by the link between seasonal foods, locally grown, home prepared, and consumed fresh has been hijacked.

What Does History Tell Us?

There are many modern enchantments that distract us from having an understanding of diet. A slanted view of human history is one of them. If we were discussing a perfect diet for any other animal aside from ourselves, we would not have the same difficulties. In discovering the healthy diet for a nonhuman, we would ask about the known history of the animal, the environment it lived in, the physical clues in the mouth and digestive system, efficiency of digestion, and even the energy requirements. We would expect these areas of inquiry to give us solid clues, and we would be right. Using these simple criteria, we would not be inclined to feed raw meat to a rabbit or porridge to a tiger. The only problem is that since it is humans who are making the decisions, enchantments come into the picture.

Humans are omnivorous; we have subsisted and even maintained health on any number of foods in our collective past. For the past several thousand years, the bulk of humanity has sustained itself on a diet of cereal grains, beans, vegetables, seeds, and fruits as the primary food. Meat, fowl, eggs, fish, and dairy products have been important components for cultures where farming was difficult or in the case where the environment or activity levels required it. As agricultural societies around the world developed, they created stability and a larger communal base. It is curious then that the image of man the hunter has played such an important role in defining our collective image of the past.

The works of writers such as Robert Ardrey and Desmond Morris popularized the notion that human aggression and violence were holdovers from our past as hunters. Their theories and a shallow reading of Darwin have had a profound effect on the way we view individual and social behavior. They have been used to explain warfare as well as many of the most unproductive elements observable in human society. They are seen as a natural outcome of the selfish gene.

While human history may be awash with violence, obstinate individualism, and aggression, the assumption that this behavior is written in our cells to be replicated as our natural way of being is cynical at best. It assumes that evolution is over. The fact that this behavior is still with us does not mean that it is essential. The rationale of man the hunter provides an easy excuse for our worst tendencies. It takes the behavior out of the realm of choice and places us in a genetic cul-de-sac with no possibility of change except through scientific intervention.

When these theories are accepted as an integral part of human nature, they become the anthropological equivalent of original sin. I have heard this argument used when objecting to vegetarian food in the form of "you need to eat meat to be strong" or "meat is man's food." I am amused by the way that some men puff out like seasoned warriors when they state that they don't eat vegetables as if it were a badge of virile masculinity.

The bones of some of our most primitive ancestors, those discovered in China and Africa, have slowly through the years been analyzed, providing a more complex picture of our origins. The image that emerges is contrary to the "hunter" thesis. There is profound evidence that the development of molars, grinding teeth, evolved through the consumption of vegetable-quality foods. The markings on the many ancient teeth are consistent with those to be expected in animals eating larger quantities of fruits, seeds, and nuts. These markings are often found without the etching that would be expected with meat eating. These conclusions, along with the high degree of manual dexterity, seem to run counter to speculation that our ancestors were primarily hunters. The evidence points to a very mixed diet that by two million years ago involved communal sharing of food, with both meat and plant foods brought to single sites to share. Since vegetables leave no bones, we must rely on the teeth and the occasional evidence of grinding stones to lead us forward.

These very ancient ancestors undoubtedly were hunters/gatherers/scavengers. They ate what was available to meet their needs for their survival. The fact that vegetable remains decompose easily and that animal bones don't is only one of the problems in interpreting primitive eating habits. There is much that is incomplete in the fossil record, and so we must also rely on common sense to inform our opinions when we use this information to inform human dietary habits.

When we see the formation of the human jaw, the arrangement of our teeth and the predominance of our cheeks, the prevalence of a meat diet seems very suspect. The incisors are useless as cutting meat fiber, the pre-molars and molars are more suited for grinding, and there are only four canine teeth. The human jaw has a fairly flat surface, not suited for tearing, more suited for grinding, and the opening to the mouth is fairly small. This small mouth opening and predominant cheeks are more suited for food that is held in the mouth and chewed rather than torn and swallowed—the habit of the carnivore. When we add this to the fact that the digestive juices in the human mouth are focused on the breakdown of complex carbohydrates, the emphasis on meat consumption as the primary source of food sounds highly questionable.

Theories of our collective evolution have an important influence on the ways in which we view ourselves and hence our vision of our future development. If we see ourselves as evolving in an environment of aggression and brutality, we accept unquestioningly and resignedly this kind of behavior when we encounter it in ourselves or in others. If, however, there is an understanding of our origins as being based on social cooperation and a sharing of resources, much can be done to influence the development of these qualities in our own society.

It needs to be said that many vegetarians use a similar exaggerated version of our shared past to put forward their case for diet and its impact on our behavior. They argue that meat eating automatically fuels the aggression and violence in society and that vegetarianism is a more sophisticated and evolved and peaceful way of nourishing ourselves. Many vegetarian cultures have long observed that the eating of meat produces aggressive and sometimes violent behavior. The problem lies in the fact that history is filled with examples of inhumanity and violence laid at the door of both vegetarians and meat eaters. History is also filled with examples of peaceful, loving people who followed just about every kind of diet imaginable. None of this contradicts the statement of Adelle Davis that "you are what you eat"; it simply makes the riddle more compelling.

The Effect of Environment

Our collective ancestry has at times relied on animal food as a primary means of sustenance. The origins of meat eating were a direct response to environmental demands including the availability of vegetable-quality foods. This is not a choice driven by preference—but of need. Simple food technology such as preserving, fermenting, drying, or making cheese from milk allowed our ancestors to create increased diversity in diet and often supplement a poor diet in the winter season. Our bodies still know when it is summer or winter, fall or spring, but we no longer meet the needs of the season, much less the area we live in.

Human diets all over the world provide a general reflection on yin and yang balance. Individuals living in a more yang climate represented by warmer weather and lower altitude are generally surrounded by a yin plant life, more abundant vegetation, and longer growing seasons. This growth provides more easily perishable vegetables, fruits, nuts, and an easier cultivation of land. A wider variety of vegetables and fruits produce a cooling yin effect on the body. Those who live in the yin colder regions with shorter growing season tend to cultivate more hearty vegetables such as roots, hearty varieties of grain, and vegetables that store well.

The variety of foods in the colder regions are scarce and cannot supply all the energy needs of human life when exposed to the climate. A colder climate dictates a greater need for fats in the diet and, depending on physical challenge, a greater need for protein. Animal fats, meat, and dairy (more yang dietary factors) will be consumed more frequently in these climates and are in balance with the yin environment. An Eskimo, living a traditional nomadic life, requires the fats and protein found in fish, seal, and other animal-source foods for good health. For a secretary spending their winters in a heated office a diet with the same protein and fat content would spell disaster. The imbalance is not simply one of quantity, but quality.

The fact that the foods found in a specific region are generally more supportive of health to those who live there should not seem strange. Like any other animal, humans must make balance with the environment they inhabit. This is a reflection of natural balance. It is reflected in the climate of a specific region as well as in the changing of the seasons. Our bodies have adapted to seasonal change since we first stood on two feet. Our bodies naturally rebel when this relationship is ignored. When we do not adapt to changes in the environment and the change of seasons, we swing out of alignment and find ourselves pulled to the extremes in an attempt to gain comfort.

I once gave a seminar in Helsinki. It was the middle of winter, and the snow was piled around the sidewalks shoulder high. The temperature was below zero, and the streets were so cold that the leather soles of my shoes were frozen into rigid planks. As I wondered around the city, I saw the bright lights of a supermarket in the distance and went to investigate. As I walked through the door, I was presented with a display featuring several cardboard palm trees and a huge mound of pineapples. Pineapples in Helsinki, what a treat! This is the story of the modern food industry, shipping tropical fruits to the frozen North so that people can undermine their health while providing ecological and economic chaos. The peculiar vision of macrobiotic thinking sees this trend not as simply fulfilling a human need for variety but an indication of our lack of consciousness regarding the food we eat.

The issue of balance is critical to environmental harmony. The most important factor in this is having a solid foundation that can be used to build on. While it is difficult for the modern world population to eat completely within the seasons on locally produced foods, adjustments can be made. These modifications are usually related to having a sensible foundation to build the diet on. In the food pyramids referred to earlier, we would notice that the healthiest diets according to international nutritional studies are based on the daily consumption of cereal grains.

Basic human needs in a temperate climate can be easily met by a grain-based diet with a good variation of vegetables, beans and bean products, seeds, nuts and fruits, sea vegetables, and a wide range of optional foods for personal needs, activity, climate, or simply enjoyment. All the essential amino acids to create protein, ample antioxidants, carbohydrate, vitamins, fats, and minerals would be present. Optional foods might include dairy foods as well as meat, fowl, fish, eggs, natural sweeteners, fruit juices, and alcoholic beverages. While some of these foods would be ignored by people on diets for special needs or shunned by some for ethical reasons, this simple dietary pattern would produce radical improvements in public health and provoke dramatic changes for the better as far as food economics is concerned.

The biggest problem is that the bulk of the modern diet is focused on the optional category. Meat, dairy, eggs, fowl, sugar, imported fruits, and vegetables as well as highly processed foods make up the bulk of the modern diet. The grain products consumed are generally grains that have been ground to flour and denatured or highly processed for quick cooking and robbed of nutritional benefit and essential fiber.

The foods in the optional category also happen to be those that lie in the extremes of yin and yang classification. They are foods with strong and often unpredictable bioenergetic effects. Because of their intense nature, they produce imbalance and the desire for extreme measures for balance. High meat and animal food consumption, extreme yang, produces heat and requires extreme yin in the form of cold foods, sugar, or alcohol. Excessive salt or food additives in the diet produce cravings for increased sweet drinks or sugar. The need of the body to produce a physical and energetic balance is in constant battle with a deluge of contradictory influences—nutritional chaos reigns. We are caught in an endless swing of the pendulum from one extreme to the other.

Cereal grains and beans store easily for long periods of time. While many nations could easily become self-sufficient in cereal production (especially with less grain fed to animals), grain and bean export and import are with us for a long time to come. Vegetables and fruit are more perishable, and so local, regional, and seasonable use is more important both for health and environmental concerns. Focus on eating locally and only using imported vegetables when needed for a healthy variety of food is a clear target. The important fact is that agriculture needs to be moved back to regional subsistence so that there is a link between the environment and the people eating the food.

In the early part of the last century, 80 percent of Americans lived on small family farms or in rural areas. During that period, a simple diet was consumed, and heart attacks were a rare cause of death. By 1930, heart attacks accounted for no more than three thousand deaths per year. Some suppose that this was because doctors at the time were unaware of the symptoms of the disease or that autopsies were not done; nothing could be further from the truth. In the 1800s, autopsies were regularly performed since it was the only way that doctors could study internal anatomy for medical research and education, nearly every dead body was a case study.

It would be absurd to imagine that our physiology, as well as our psychology, was not greatly influenced by the quality and type of foods we choose in our evolutionary journey. For thousands of years, these patterns continued with very little deviation as a result of our natural adaptation to the environment. If we agree that the wonderful development of the human body and brain were influenced by specific dietary practices, we should be very cautious of abrupt changes. The diversity of the human diet is certainly reflected in the diversity of our capabilities. But that diversity has had a close relationship to the specific environments that we inhabited at various stages of our development. This fact of environmental approach to diet has not been investigated much at all. Making assumptions about the role of food in human evolution have limited importance if not guided by some principle that can include the arc of human development including the development of agriculture.

The evolutionary past, the path of our ancestors, requires a particular biological resonance. If we want to reclaim our health, we must replicate the energy that brought us to our present state of evolution, but with a new consciousness. One of the things that can be brought forward is the respect for the source of our being, and our diet plays an important role in bringing that respect to the fore. If our diet does not respect the needs of the planet, then it will produce illness. We become strangers to the earth.

A Macrobiotic View of Food Energies

The use of yin and yang qualities of food provides a useful complement to the science of nutrition. It is user friendly since the qualities described are ones that can be perceived clearly by the individual. We don't usually hear a person "experience" a protein or a mineral, but we can easily learn to experience the effects of different foods.

The perception of these energies is a learned life skill. They are the qualities of feelings, intuition, as well as observation, self-awareness, and common sense. It is here that the accumulated wisdom of our ancestry can be of the greatest help since the road maps and operating manuals for further developing these capacities within ourselves have been well delineated by the sages, philosophers, and wise men and women of the past. It may well be one of the most important tasks facing our modern civilization: to blend these insights and experiences with the materialistic and scientific observations of the last several centuries. One of the fascinating aspects of using this philosophy is how the conclusions of this primitive way of thinking are so closely aligned with the most recent suggestions on diet by health researchers.

The dietary practices recommended by Michio Kushi in the 1980s as the standard macrobiotic diet were an attempt to return to more traditional eating patterns. The emphasis on the consumption of grains, beans, vegetables, nuts and seeds, and variety of supplemental foods to balance individual needs certainly was a step in the right direction. It was a call to return to some semblance of natural order in nutrition so that we could move forward, motivated by health rather than profit. His diet proved effective for tens of thousands of men and women who were suffering from poor health. It has a direct influence on our biological integrity and behavior since it reduces stress resulting from the consumption of foods that challenge our biological integrity.

Thousands of people used the macrobiotic approach to reclaim their health after diagnosis with a wide range of diagnosed illness. Many of those using the diet with positive effect had cancer, and the diet became increasingly known as a diet for the treatment of that disease. Motivated by fear, many who followed the diet applied it in the most restrictive way, leading to a perception that the macrobiotic way of eating was a stringent approach to diet and difficult to follow. Over time, common sense has triumphed over dogma, and the simplicity and flexibility of macrobiotics has emerged.

If we see foods as part of the continuing process of nature, we can observe that plants and animals all have unique qualities and characteristics. Some of these qualities can be described through analysis, but many only become apparent by observing relationships within the total environment. How plants grow, when they ripen, where they come from, when their seeds or fruits are mature, how they have been traditionally used and in some cases their biological purpose. These are simple measures of what it is that we are eating.

A good example of this is the use of milk. Traditionally, milk was used in areas where vegetable-quality food was scarce or during the winter months. Since there was no ability to store these products for long periods of time, milk was often fermented or made into cheese for later use. The animals producing them were usually few; consumption levels per person were normally low.

The "biological purpose" of milk is to nurture the young of a particular species. Nutritional requirements vary from one mammal to the next. The specific requirements for a calf are a direct response to the necessity for fast bone growth so that the young calf can stand quickly and stay with the herd. The milk is "designed" to promote rapid bone growth.

The emphasis of growth in a human baby is more concentrated on the development of the nervous system and brain. There is not the need for a rapid increase in size. (The baby does not learn to stand and walk until many months after birth.) This simple observation concerning the qualities of a particular food should give us pause for thought. There is a specific underlying order in nature that often defies analysis. When we perceive that there is an order in nature, we realize that it is important to cooperate with this order to create personal health and stability.

This way of thinking lies at the basis of traditional folk medicine and is reflected in the contemporary view of macrobiotic philosophy. If we can better understand these qualitative factors, it will be helpful in understanding the effects of foods on our health, perception, thought, and action. The philosophy of yin and yang provides us with the basis for seeing these qualities more clearly. We can discover practical ways to create a balance between the environment and ourselves. Foods such as meat, sugar, dairy food, and modern/processed foods all have specific effects on the body and mind which are a direct result not only of their nutritional value but also of the energetic qualities that they possess. The same is true of grains, vegetables, and all foods. While every food has both yin and yang components, one factor will dominate in the way they affect us.

Cereal grains are generally put at the center of the spectrum of foods due to their usefulness in combining with other foods as a dietary foundation. The cereals are the primary food for the planet. They are yang in that they are compact and complete; being both the seed and fruit of the plant, they are dried and stored so that they can be used all year round. They are yin in their profusion with hundreds of grains on one plant. Ohsawa often used the motto One Grain, Ten Thousand Grains to indicate the mentality of a healthy individual, multiplying the gift of life in the way that one seed of rice can produce such abundance. The whole cereal grains represent the fulcrum that most macrobiotic diets would be based on, depending on specific environmental needs.

The complement to whole grains in most cultures are beans. They are found in many varieties and have been used for centuries as the perfect complement to grains. They are more yin than the grains; they are also the seed and fruit of the plant but are larger, more porous, and contain a higher amount of oil. Beans come in many varieties and range from the smaller more yang beans such as aduki beans and lentils to the yin larger beans such as soy or lima beans. Long cooking or fermentation to improve digestion and liberate their nutritional benefits have been traditionally used in Africa and Asia, Europe and the Americas.

The term *vegetables* covers a wide variety of edible leafs, stems, and roots that have been used in traditional cooking. Compared to beans and grains, they are more yin as a group being softer in structure, more perishable, and containing a higher percentage of water. Some of these are more dominated by yin energy and some by yang. The broad leafy vegetables are more yin, and root vegetables are more yang. A good variety of vegetables is essential for a healthy diet, containing both roots and leaves as well as comprising vegetables of different colors—a sign recently discovered to indicate the presence of antioxidants.

In terms of seasons of growth and place of origin, foods originating in colder climates have a tendency to be more yang, and those originating in warm or tropical climates tend to be more yin. Fruits such as apples, pears, and berries are more cool climate fruits and more yang as opposed to tropical fruits such as mango, papaya, or pineapple that have more yin characteristics such as sugars and acids.

In more traditional forms of medicine, the characteristics of plant growth and, in fact, animal behavior were seen as indications of the way consumption of these foods would affect the person eating them. It was a literal interpretation of that statement, "You are what you eat." This theory was applied actively in the treatment of both physical and emotional imbalances. If an individual exhibited physical symptoms or behavior that were more expansive or diffuse by nature, then foods classified at the other end of the spectrum as being more compacted and concentrated would be suggested to stimulate internal harmony. If, on the other hand, a person was rigid and inflexible and showed the physical or mental symptoms of excessive yang, those foods identified with promoting relaxation and expansion would be used.

An example of this would be the use of the mushroom, an extremely yin food. There are hundreds of kinds of mushrooms, many with exceptional healing properties. The kind normally used in America and in Europe is the white button mushrooms. The yin character of these is easily seen in the fact that if rubbed vigorously, they fragment—they have form, but little substance. It is as if it were an illusion. The plant was quite commonly used in folk medicine for people who were tight, irritable, or overly rigid in their behavior and thinking. Some mushrooms have such extreme yin qualities that they were used in shamanic practices in Siberia, in Mexico by native priest-healers, and in Europe for their psychoactive properties.

We can also look at foods from an animal source with the same perspective. All meat, fish, fowl, or mammal is seen as being on the yang end of the spectrum.

There is, however, a distinction made between the type of yang and that seen in the vegetable kingdom. The Chi has been realigned to the animal source and been permeated with that creature's innate qualities. Macrobiotic suggestions regarding use of animal-source foods generally stress eating lower on the food chain and selecting those creatures that are more primitive if flesh foods are used.

Among the fish, the faster-moving fish or those with red meat are more yang while the slower-moving fish, generally with white meat, are more yin. Among the fowl, wild birds are more active and yang while cultivated birds are more yin. Among mammals, the red meat animal (that is wild is less fatty and remain in their natural state) are most yang as compared to domesticated or slow-moving animals. In the following chapters, there is more discussion of the avoidance or use of different foods.

In terms of both Western nutrition and Eastern medicine's energetic classifications of food, balance is essential. This means realizing that there are complementary relationships both in terms of specific nutrients and energetic qualities that must be established in order for the body to function at its highest potential.

In macrobiotics, the various qualities of yin and yang are used to identify the character of foods so that proper balance can be achieved. If we see that one particular group of foods has a predominant influence in affecting the body in a particular way, it is helpful for us to know which foods provide the opposite effect so that a diet can be created that reduces the stresses caused by extremes. Understanding these classifications is important not only in terms of daily food consumption and the preparation of meals but also in redressing long-standing imbalances in the individual's condition.

Through proper food selection and preparation, we are consciously assisting the body rather than assuming that the body will work everything out on its own. The point is not to become obsessed with food selection, but to reeducate it so that the distinction between what nourishes, what harms, and what is simply a sensory treat become apparent. When this process is underway, the act of eating food that serves us becomes an intuitive act and not an intellectual riddle or an obsessive dogma.

Chapter Ten

Body and Mind

A Personal Odyssey

Shortly after my introduction to macrobiotics, I had my first insight into the power that food has on perception. I went on a weeklong camping trip into the mountains around the Little Sur River on the California coast. I though it would be interesting to experiment with my diet and so only took some grains, a few vegetables, and tea with me. I had been attempting to follow macrobiotic principles in my eating for several months but was not especially disciplined in my practice. I found that avoiding meat and dairy were easy and that only sugar posed a problem. It seemed to me that being alone in the woods, beyond temptation, was a perfect place to test the claims of Ohsawa regarding the power of dietary simplicity.

After spending a day packing into the mountains, I set up camp beside a stream and cooked up my first meal. The food tasted unusually good, but that's always been my experience in the mountains. I hiked, sat by the river, meditated, chewed rice, and read. The mountains had never looked, smelled, or felt better—even the night it rained. In all my years of camping out and being alone in nature, I had never felt so close to the wilderness that surrounded me. After two days, the vegetables were gone, and I decided to soldier on. I was simply eating rice and buckwheat sprinkled with sesame seeds and drinking tea—fairly close to what Ohsawa described as a rice fast. When my food ran out, I hiked back to the coast, got in my car, and drove back to San Francisco. I felt wonderful.

When I arrived home, I felt like an alien from another planet. My perception of my surroundings was definitely altered. This was the sixties, and so I was no stranger to altered perception, but this was very different. I was aware of a heightened state of sensory awareness unlike anything I had experienced before. This went beyond my usual comparison between the crisp and clean lines of nature and the oily, hard surfaces of the city. It was not a good/bad distinction; it was simply a deeper sense of reality.

As I continued my macrobiotic experiment in San Francisco, I began to notice other changes as well. The anxious nature that had dominated my youth and teens seemed to drift into the background. I felt calmer, happier, and more in control of my life than I had ever felt. The drugs that had served as my exit strategy from unhappiness now seemed unattractive. As my physical health improved, my emotional life became more harmonious. There was no question for me that my diet and my improved health were the reasons I felt more peaceful and alert.

In later years, as I began to teach the macrobiotic philosophy and coach people in their practice, I continued to see the same emotional response in clients and students. Since many of the people who came to me for counseling had physical problems, the changes in their emotional life were an unexpected bonus. My clients consistently commented on the sense of calmness and clarity that accompanied their shift in diet. It was these comments that inspired me to study the principles of the Five Transformations from Chinese medicine and later to publish *Macrobiotics and Human Behavior* in 1984.

In that book, I outlined my reflections on how the Chinese system of the Five Transformations was used to gain insight into the connection between physical health and behavior. This way of looking at the effect of daily actions on health and the effect of specific organ functions on behavior is fascinating. While based on the vision of health as the relationship between the individual and the environment, it presents the potential for incorporating modern insights regarding the way that family, culture, and biological influences combine to affect sensitivity and response to the world around us. It also implies an interesting link between the food we eat and how we act.

Food, Blood, and Brain

The story of our individual lives is the sum total of our biology, culture, and spiritual awareness. We are influenced, for better or worse, by our food, environment, and the mysterious process of our own particular interpretation of the experiences that life has placed in our path. It is intriguing to imagine that we can pick one specific event or stimulus that governs who we are and why we respond to life the way we do, but that is probably a fool's game.

I have met those who were raised in the most abject poverty or suffered from the most horrible abuse and were compassionate and inspiring people. I have met men and women who have dealt with major afflictions of the body and were successful and happy. The opposite is also true. Happy environments, affection, and careful nurturing do not always produce saints.

Of all the various factors that shape our lives, it is interesting that the influence of health on our behavior is often laid to the side except in the case of gross imbalances in brain chemistry. This is especially true when considerations of diet enter the picture. Unless we are discussing the dramatic effect of a particular food additive or chemical pollutant on the mind, the power of what we eat is thought to be a superficial and eccentric consideration. If we know that food affects health, why not take that fact to the next level of consideration. While the implication that food can be the unique cause for all emotional distress or destructive behavior is ill advised. It is true that what we eat affects our awareness and our state of total being. _

At the most superficial level of experience, we all know that if we have a cold, a stomach upset, or a headache, we behave differently toward the world around us. That world includes the people as well as the car that refuses to start, or the computer that is slow in booting up. We may become irritable and short-tempered or vulnerable—we are not our usual cheerful self. We are aware that our physiology is promoting a difference in the way we respond. Many people are aware that when they drink too much coffee, they become a twitching, nervous wreck, but what if they accept that as simply "the way they are"?

How we describe normal is the issue. We all perceive the world through our own lens. We all act out of that perception and have learned ways of reacting to the world around us. This habitual way of experiencing and acting in the world is our own personal normal. If we are not self-critical, we accept this state as a given. I get angry because "that's just the way I am"; maybe I procrastinate because "I have always been that way." It is easy to simply accept a pattern of behavior, a habit of action, when it defines who we are. It is difficult to see the foundation of these habits, how they may inhibit our growth, if we are not able to experience a different perspective. If the driving force of the habit is subtle and not immediately associated with an unusual symptom or obvious indulgence, it may escape us completely. It is in this realm that the relationship between what we eat and how we act is most interesting.

The brain is the most sensitive organ in the body to minute changes in the chemistry of the blood. There is a complex and little understood phenomenon called the blood-brain barrier that is designed to protect the brain from dangerous toxicity. While the rest of the capillaries in the body allow soluble chemicals to pass through, the cells that make up the capillaries of the brain are more tightly packed. This structure only allows certain molecules entrance. This is why the brain is protected from most infections and why treatment of many physiological problems that occur in the brain are difficult to treat with drugs—the brain doesn't allow the drugs access.

The problem with all of this is that we well know that many natural substances that affect the function of the brain gain access quite easily. The psychoactive molecules of marijuana, alcohol, and many mind-altering drugs seem to have no problem at all. After decades of study, the actual mechanism of how these chemicals alter perception is still not understood. It is not difficult to see why something as subtle as changes in blood chemistry as a result of diet cannot be measured and registered if there is no real understanding of the ways that the psychological juggernaut of LSD is a mystery.

The physical aspect of this relationship seems very simple. Air, water, and food are taken into the body by respiration and digestion. The absorbed nutrients are then assembled to create the cells of the body and blood. The blood circulates through the body and nourishes the cells of body including the brain and carries away the residue of cellular activity to be excreted. The quality of these nutritive factors is known to have a profound effect on the health of the organs and tissue of the body. We know that these nutritional factors affect the rise of most degenerative diseases, but what about the brain? Is it somehow exempt from this simple and elegant circulation of nutrients? It is a simple act of logic to know that what we eat affects our brain function. The only question is how.

When I was in India, I met a gentleman who had a lifetime of migraine headaches that caused him to be irritable and abrupt with his family and friends. He had traveled the world, trying to find a cure. During a conversation with a friend and I, we boldly said that he could probably rid himself of the condition if he changed his diet. He was interested in our strange ideas and invited us to stay with him in Bombay and advise his cook. After several weeks, the headaches were gone. With the pain went the irritability. We were never able to stop him referring to us as his "American Doctors." For him, it was a simple process. It's not always that easy, but we never know till we try.

Mind/Body—Body and Mind

The Western scientific model has focused on the material aspects of cell functioning, tissue groupings, organ systems, and gross anatomy. The Eastern approach has placed more emphasis on attempting to understand the underlying energetic reality. It is not necessary to attempt to link this energetic reality to modern physics as is often done. The phenomenon of felt energy is something we perceive daily. We are built to do this, and it is only the fact that we do not know how to nurture this faculty and use it creatively that we understand it poorly. All matter—including the body—is composed of energy. Distinctions perceived in material phenomena bear a direct relationship to the "frequency" of the energies involved in their creation.

The observation of a life force was of course not limited to the Chinese. The medicine of ancient India called it prana, the Japanese called it ki, and scores of ancient traditions on every continent discussed this energy. Concepts of life force energy continue to form the basis of many alternative approaches to healing and often referred to as *bioenergetic energy* (a term also used in conventional medicine regarding energy exchanges on the molecular level and in the work of Alexander Lowen and disciples of Wilhelm Reich). It is good to note that for many scientists, these theories are the work of heretics. I include the following quote from a published article by Victor J. Stenger, Department of Physics and Astronomy at the University of Hawaii:

> **If bioenergetic fields exist, then some two hundred years of physics, chemistry, and biology has to be re-evaluated .... It is one thing to publish a low significance result that does not violate known principles; it is another to publish one that forces science to undergo a paradigm-shift and redirect the limited resources of research to areas that are extremely unlikely to produce any pay-off.**

With apologies to Mr. Stenger, "the risk of re-evaluating 200 years of physics, chemistry and biology" seems a small price to pay compared to the vast store of wisdom in Chinese medicine with a recorded history of over four thousand years and the Ayurvedic system of India that represents at least three thousand years of written history. This is especially true when we consider that these systems stand for centuries of experience prior to being written. They reflect observations made on millions of people, not studies done on several hundred. It is fully accepted that the Chinese and Indians developed the most extensive and accurate natural pharmacopoeias ever assembled. Why then should we look away from the way that the discoveries were made?

The analysis of the human body described in Chinese medicine is vastly different than the one we are used to. As in many other cultures, the body is seen as an energy field in constant interaction with the environment. The sophisticated understanding that they demonstrated regarding the function and structure of the physical organs, the development of disease process and human behavior were all observed to reflect this constant movement of energy. This is vision that sees the body as permeable to the energy that enlivens it.

The energy that we take in the form of physically measurable substance such as air, water, and food comprise only a part of our bioenergetic needs. The response to our environment overlaps the edge of physical measurement and the feeling state. We know that being in forests, near streams, or at the seashore make most people relaxed. This effect is often placed at the door of negative ions that are abundant in air at these places, but is that the extent of the influence?

Ancient peoples and many indigenous cultures still intact know that there are certain places in nature that have beneficent aspects that can stimulate physical, emotional, and spiritual states. They may be springs that contain healing waters, rock formations that stimulate meditative states, or any particular configuration in the landscape. When confronted with these natural fields of Chi, the effect is visceral. The energy of the space permeates our being and nourishes us. The same phenomenon may take place in conversation with a person or exposure to a piece of music. The energy of the person or event holds the potential to nurture us in a way that is not measurable by science, but still deeply felt.

The Asian cultures reflected and recorded these effects in great detail for centuries. They also studied the ways that Chi moved through the body in a complex series of energetic pathways called the meridians. These channels of energy flow still form the basis for acupuncture treatment thousands of years after their discovery and defy the scientific methods used to attempt to rationalize them even by the doctors in hospitals where they are used as treatment.

There are conflicting viewpoints as to how our primitive ancestors arrived at this seemingly sophisticated point of view without the existence of extensive technologies. Their capacity to perceive an energetic reality beneath the surface of the material world has been ascribed to latent mystical powers of insight, fortuitous accident, and even to the existence of technologies thousands of years ago of which we are not aware. It is more likely that their conclusions regarding the true nature of the world were simply a logical outcome of the fact that they dealt directly with the changing patterns of nature and learned to hone their sensitivity to them. If our lives depend on being able to read the signs of the earth, to know when to plant, when to harvest, when the rains will come, or when the cold winds will blow, then we are certainly placed in a position where the inherent patterns and order of the environment will reveal themselves.

These ancient observers did not simply invent an arbitrary set of rules for human use; they experienced themselves as part of the continuum of nature. Without romanticizing their culture or habits, it is easy to see that if we take away all the trappings of the built environment, we would have a different view of the world we lived in. They created a language that was rich with a symbolism that allowed a more complete exploration of various energy states and how those energies transformed and mutated in environmental process and in human life. Having concepts that describe energy that is felt but not seen allows conversations to take place that would otherwise be impossible. The language of these traditional forms of spiritual philosophy and medicine is a language filled with metaphor and allusion. It is the language of poetry, not of science—it is also the language of human experience.

Within this model, the body is perceived as a community of cells that all work together to produce the state of health and vitality. The organ systems of the body are perceived as each being home to a particular quality of energy that is essential to the welfare of the whole. What we observe in this approach is a vision of health governed by an internal ecology. This view has to do with the natural relationship between the organs and organ systems. Some of the descriptions of organic function imagine the relationships between the organs as an internal government with various departments.

Each organ system or department has a particular biological function that is based on its energetic character. The degree of cooperation between these departments defines health and the way in which the total organism responds to the challenges of existence. The big surprise is that the brain, the organ we consider to be the pinnacle of human uniqueness, doesn't even get a seat at the table.

Each member of this committee needs a particular kind of nourishment in order to function at its highest level in order to contribute to the whole. The nourishment essential for the effective function of the internal government comes in many forms. All of the basic needs discussed in earlier chapters are required, but the functioning of perception, reaction, and response are a reflection of the overall balance of the body and not placed as the exclusive domain of one organ. The Chinese had a very sophisticated understanding or physiology and knew the brain was there. They simply saw the function of that organ as reflecting the health of the whole system.

Five Phases of Change

As energy moves from yin to yang in the cycle of expansion to contraction, it exhibits different qualities and characteristics. The Chinese observed five distinct phases in this process. They labeled each phase with a corresponding phenomenon in nature. These phases of energy are not separate—each phase feeds the next. This cycle of movement is generally referred to as the five transformations theory or the five elements theory.

The terms used to describe these qualities are *soil, metal, water, tree,* and *fire*. These terms should not be interpreted in a literal sense. They are metaphors for qualities of energy that are observable in nature. If yin and yang are the rhythm in the symphony of nature, the five transformations are the notes in the scale.

While this system is used to describe many phenomena in nature and human society, I am limiting the discussion to the health and behavior relationship. Each phase of development in this transformation cycle is essential for the next phase to be nourished. The effectiveness of energy to manifest itself in each successive phase is dependent upon how effectively the energy has moved to the full potential in the one preceding.

Imagine a circle on the right side the energy is descending, first loosely then more contracted. This side is the yang aspect of the cycle and represented by the soil and metal stages. As the energy moves across the bottom and up the left side, it expands back our and then rises. This upward or yin part of the cycle is represented in the water and tree stages. At the top of the circle, energy is dispersed out of the circle and drawn back in, this is the fire phase of energy. The energy drawn back into the circle moves down toward soil. It is helpful to imagine the characteristics of each phase as symbols of the natural phenomena represented.

The Image of Soil—Soil energy can be seen as the first stage of the contracting yang movement. It represents settling, nourishing a gentle downward motion. The image of the forest floor where all matter is decomposed. The top layer of the soil is soft and decaying and rich in life and activity. As it settles deeper, it becomes more concentrated and firm. This settling process leads to the next stage of transformation—metal.

The Image of Metal—The metal stage is the most completely yang of the five stages. It is energy at the greatest state of concentration. This is the stage where energy is most compact and densely composed. An image often associated with this is the image of ore or stone. When energy is tightly compressed, it seeks expansion. The potential of metal energy finds its release in water.

The Image of Water—This stage describes the release of dynamic tension as outward movement. The image of water indicates the viscous qualities inherent in the beginnings of this movement. Water is relentless in its movement, always seeking, always in motion. Rain falls upon the earth and flows into lakes, rivers, and streams, moving continually toward the sea.

The Image of Tree—The movement of water in its stage of evaporation is closely aligned with the energetic qualities described in tree energy. Here the Chi is ascending. It is the impulse behind the growth of plants upward and toward the sun, the rising energy of morning mists, and any movement up and away from the surface of the planet. At this stage, Yin loses some of the spontaneity of water and becomes more ordered, channeled, and defined in its movement.

The Image of Fire—The image of fire is analogous to the sun and to the fire of the hearth. It can warm and comfort or be fierce in its blaze. It provides heat and warmth as well as consuming what fuels it.

The circulation of Chi through the body takes on the character of these energies, and each phase must be nourished in order for health to manifest. These qualities are only aspects of the one primal flow; the individual qualities require specific nourishment so that health can be maintained in the system. It is the balance of these qualities that produce the greatest potential for the state of authentic self to emerge.

Each stage of transformation has biological, emotional, and spiritual qualities that can be animated by a harmonious balance within the cycle. If the various stages of transformation are allowed to complete themselves, the individual's capacity for maintaining a healthy existence is enhanced. If, however, the energies are blocked, stagnated, or if any particular phase becomes overly excited, then the effect of the energies become perverse, producing ill health, disharmony, tension, or confusion.

This theory establishes a direct relationship between those biochemical and energetic events occurring within the physical body and their corresponding effect on our abilities to perceive and act effectively. It points to the direct relationship between blood quality and brain function, which also provides for our evolving understanding of the energetic qualities that lie beneath the surface of the material world. In Asian medicine, the understanding of this cycle and the results of disruption in it are the basis of both physical and emotional diagnosis as well as the type of treatment required.

In the healing arts, a very sophisticated understanding of this process is essential for the treatment of serious illness. That does not mean that the system is limited to professional use. The understanding of how our health affects our action and perception can be an important tool for creating a balanced life. The health and personal transformation suggestions in the following chapters fall into that category. The treatment of specific disorders lies outside the scope of this book.

Every aspect of our life experience affects the cycle of energy. What we eat, our emotional experiences, our environment, the air we breathe, our culture, and the water we drink all either stress or dissipate our bioenergetic state. The events and actions of our life may stimulate or stagnate our potential. The puzzle of personal health and authenticity can be greatly helped by an appreciation of this simple view of the nature of life. This cycle of energy is not completely dictated by any one factor. In the next chapter, I will put forward a view of how the cycle of change can be used to better understand our personal, physical, and emotional well-being.

Chapter Eleven

Five Archetypes

The Internal Landscape

One thing that unifies all human life on the planet is our impulse to create stories. We create stories about our place in the world, how the world works, the limits of our personal capacities and why we are the way we are. Those stories are a powerful tool we use to have the world make sense. We all do it, I do it, you do it; every leader in politics, religion, and science does it. There are even stories about how stories are dangerous, but they are still stories. We give stories weight and importance, depending on who tells them, where we hear or read them, how they are communicated, and if they fit our definition of what a good story should be. Do we classify the story as fact or fiction? This question is only answerable by comparison to the most fascinating story of all—our myth of being—our masterpiece. Since I am going to be using this term, I want to be clear about my meaning.

A myth can be seen as a story about heroes and supernatural beings or simply as a fable or a fairy tale; it may even be called a lie. The self-created story of our life is not simply a factual and chronological account of what happened to us. It is fashioned by our view of those thoughts, emotions, and events and our interpretation of them. It is usually informed by the enchantments of our culture. The characters and happenings in our personal story take on symbolic meaning to us. It is the story that serves as the standard that all other information must conform to.

Our myth of being is a story woven with threads of body, mind, and spirit. It will contain strands manufactured through education, religion, or personal experience. It depends on cultural values of gender, race, and social standing. It provides the backdrop and setting for all our internal dialogue, the self-talk that goes on endlessly, for better or worse, as we repair, reinforce, or dismantle parts of the story that don't seem to fit the moment. The myth of being may spur us forward or hold us back.

A question here might be why a particular person is more or less receptive to a particular myth of being. We know that simply because a person has the same parents, is raised in the same culture, and educated in the same school, they will not have the same leanings as a brother or sister. Genetics or education does not seem to be consistent in swaying aesthetic sensibilities, political passions, or religious fervor. There is much talk about the importance of developing a healthy internal dialogue, a topic in the following chapter, but even that internal dialogue exists within our unique perception and experience. This filtering mechanism is our character—that set of qualities that make us distinct from other people.

Throughout history, it has been observed people can be classified into character types. These categories of behavior were sometimes seen as the result of astrological influences, physiology, or combinations of any number of material or supernatural forces. The Greeks undoubtedly had the most influence on the modern practice of personality typing. Hippocrates classified four distinct humors relative to the health of his patients. By AD 200, Galen concluded that the humors influenced personality as well as health. He concluded that phlegm promoted calm behavior where excess blood produced the cheerful sanguine personality; bile was associated with depression, and choleric types were hot tempered.

Contemporary versions of personality typing are the PSI (personal style indicator) and Myers-Briggs methods that are used in present-day business. The Myers-Briggs test is used by many businesses to match the best candidates for jobs and to assist people to better understand their distinctive abilities in pursuing vocations. The most recent and accepted classifications are the so-called Big Five (BF) system that was developed by two independent teams of researchers.

The model was first presented to the American Psychological Association in 1933. Later studies by Paul Costa and Robert McCrae at the National Institutes of Health and Warren Norman (University of Michigan) and Lewis Goldberg (University of Oregon) used different routes in arriving at startlingly similar conclusions. They discovered that human personality could be defined in five dimensions regardless of culture. They were able to make this classification through interviews with thousands of people. They did not set out to prove the correlations; the connections emerged from their findings.

One of the main problems with any system that attempts to explain our personality type is that that there are many events that contribute to our character. Whatever system we use is only helpful if there is a flexibility that allows other factors of potential influence to intervene. Life is dynamic, changing, and filled with the unexpected. We all have the capacity to change and the ability to take advantage of our unique talents and improve our shortcomings. When we cling fiercely to an explanation of our nature, we give away the ability to pursue our personal transformation. A primary challenge is to discover tools that personalize the process. This does not rely on therapists, doctors, gurus, or mediums—it is dependent on being able to judge through experience the cause and effect of our actions.

I have found the Five Transformation system in Chinese medicine fascinating both in my personal life and in my observations and work with clients over the years. This system points to an interesting link between the physical, emotional, mental, and spiritual aspects of our being. It is used as a diagnostic tool by practitioners but is perhaps most useful as a personal guidebook. Unfortunately much that is written in on the character types has to do with classification of pathologies. I have favored descriptions that are aimed at the personal rather than the clinical use.

These Five Archetypes do not describe any single person, but they apply to everyone. As one psychologist said of the BF system, "It is the psychology of the stranger." They are easily recognized, but usually exclude much of the internal life of a person. A distinguishing factor of the Chinese system is that it comments on both the positive as well as the shadow aspects of each character type and links those obvious characteristics with personal health and insights to the nourishing or tempering of imbalances.

In the Five Transformations Cycle, each stage of energetic movement has its own characteristics. When the full cycle of transformation is permitted to complete itself, a consistent pattern of regeneration is present as Chi energy vitalizes the cells and tissue of the body. When the energies are blocked, then the qualities turn back on themselves. The disharmony present in a blocked situation creates physical or psychological characteristics that are contradictory to the process of transformation, and a course of energetic degeneration sets in.

Symptoms presenting themselves both physically or emotionally can be classified within this system and used to form a comprehensive picture of an individual's overall state of health. The advantage of this approach to diagnosis is not merely the classification of symptoms, but also the ability to see problems in their early stages. Common to other forms of Oriental diagnosis the object is to see early signs of imbalance rather than wait for more serious symptoms to appear. Once a problem is identified, steps can be taken to make corrections in the individual's way of life, which can bring about a reversal of the illness or at least prevent its further development. As a tool for personal growth, it provides the individual with information that he or she can use to assist in the creation of improved health and stability.

This chapter presents the general characteristics observable in both the positive and negative phases of energy transformation. It also describes the ways in which these energetic imbalances affect general characteristics of behavior—gesture, posture, and other forms of body language. Recreating our bond with Gaia requires a transformative process from each of us. What better place to learn the from the transformations of energy that take place daily in nature. I have included some ideas as to the physiological basis of this approach as well as some suggestions for regaining balance. One thing that is helpful to keep in mind is that, like any system that attempts to provide insight or reasons for what we do, the system can be abused.

My grandfather used to say, "If it's not broke, don't fix it." The emotional states described as symptoms of imbalance are only significant if they dominate a person's existence. Anger, depression, self-pity, or any number of emotional experiences move in and out of our lives. I believe them to be natural and even healthy. I would think that someone who is never angry or has never been depressed or experienced self-pity was unusual.

The Five Energy Archetypes

Compassion/Settling (Soil)

Positive Character Attributes

The positive attributes of the soil character are perceived as one of the most balanced stages in the cycle of energy. They describe the settling quality of yang energy. It represents stability, resourcefulness, and the capacity for steady perseverance. We may say that they are solid, grounded, or have their feet planted solidly on the earth.

When soil energy is healthy in an individual there is a feeling of satisfaction and stability. It is out of this feeling that compassion arises. When we feel stable and self-reliant, our ability to reach out and assist others is enhanced. The feeling of internal resourcefulness makes it possible for the individual to be generous since they have no internal doubt as to their own capacities.

In the BF system this type is called "agreeable." They cite the qualities of being interested in others, willing to take time out to listen to others, and to sympathize with other peoples' emotions. They are seen to be generous with their time and energy.

The description of this phase corresponds to the PSI type referred to as "solid." This style is generally described as peace loving, quiet, and avoiding conflict. In some interpretations of the PSI, they are called "friends" or "supporters." The description found in Chinese medicine, the BF and the PSI, are perfectly in line.

The Shadow Character of Soil

The Big Five system seems to place dysfunctional aspects of character in a single type. The PSI only comments on the positive aspects of character; this limits the usefulness of these models since the one places all problems in one type and the other does not relate to any problems at all. When this energy is blocked or becomes stagnated, those exact qualities that identify the character type turn in on themselves. Cheerfulness turns to complaining, compassion turns to self-pity or jealousy, and trust turns to suspicion. The sense of physical resilience drifts toward anxiety regarding health and well-being.

Instead of giving compassion, they seek compassion. They complain about their state of health, the incapacity of others to fulfill their needs, and the insensitivity of the world at large. Their self-image is often that of the victim. In their relationships with others, they are apt to be frustrated. Since they are continually seeking reassurance, others may become impatient with their demands and try to avoid contact with them. They sincerely desire warmth and close contact with others, and rejection can produce in them feelings of suspicion and cynicism. They are prone to falling into the view that hypocrisy rules. In its extreme, depleted soil energy can produce feelings of jealousy and martyrdom.

These feelings are not based on any conscious process or attempt toward the manipulation of others. The behavior can only be understood by ascribing a type of reactive consciousness to the organism as a whole. The individuals are simply seeking some way to fill what they feel is a growing need. Unconsciously, they may even place themselves in difficult situations that are sure to elicit the sympathy and/or pity of others.

Physical Characteristics and Habits

Physically, there are certain tendencies that are common to the ailments brought about by frustrated or depleted soil energy. There is a tendency for the muscles to become flaccid. This is especially true of the lower limbs. There is a tendency to hold weight in the lower part of the body in the buttocks and thighs. The flaccidity of the muscles can often be seen most strikingly in the face. The features lack sharp definition, and there is a tendency for slackness in facial expression.

There is a peculiarity in gesture, which can be characterized as non-completion. Hand gestures often begin and then simply dissipate, with hands falling to the side or in the lap. The hands often seem heavy and show little or no expressive grace. The gestures and speech often reflect a state of futility. A characteristic of the voice is often a plaintive. They may punctuate their conversation with sighs.

Meridian Energy

Disharmony in the spleen and stomach creates imbalances in the corresponding acupuncture meridians in the legs. The effect of this is usually weakness in the legs, especially in climbing or pushing, and a decrease in the circulation of blood. This often contributes to a feeling of heaviness in the lower part of the body and flaccidity in the muscles of the inner thigh. The person often has a sense of limited "push," which undermines endurance. This energetic imbalance contributes to the tendency to put on and hold weight.

Physiological Considerations

In Oriental medicine, soil energy is perceived as the energy that animates the functioning of the spleen and pancreas and the stomach. The spleen has as one of its primary functions the storage of blood, which is called forth as the body's demands increase. It also functions as part of the lymphatic system necessary for the body to protect itself from infection as part of the immune system. The spleen is a storage place for formed elements extracted from damaged blood cells, saving them for later use. All of these are resource functions, providing a general backup system for the body as needed. When the body loses its ability to protect and strengthen, we become cautious in much the same way that we will favor or protect a damaged arm or leg when wounded. We become wary of the world around us.

The pancreas, on the other hand, serves as a primary control over the blood sugar level, which is a control of the body's resources of stored energy. If we attribute a degree of cellular consciousness to the organism, we see that the body can perceive the lack of resources and inability to meet immediate energy needs. In this scenario, the individuals lack the confidence to extend themselves fully, feel that they must conserve what they have and compels them to rely on others for their needs. A common theme in the myth of being for this type includes the need for help or rescue.

Contributing Factors

There are many factors that can exacerbate imbalances in soil. Two of these are nutrition and emotional experience. Regarding the influence of food, one of the most powerful negatives is the consumption of refined sugar. Refined sugar and any simple sugar in the diet can put unusual stress on the pancreas as well as robbing the body of mineral stores that are so essential in immune function. Since the natural qualities of soil energy promote stability and the nurturing of resources, the effect of simple sugars undermines this by leaching energy and resources from the body.

In the last twenty years, we have increased sugar consumption in the America from twenty-six pounds to one hundred thirty-five pounds of sugar per person per year. Before the turn of this century (1887-1890), the average consumption was only five pounds per person per year. Highly refined sugars such as white sugar, brown sugar, corn sugar, and high-fructose corn syrup are being used in many foods such as breakfast cereal, peanut butter, ketchup, sauces, and a wide variety of processed foods. They are especially high in foods specifically designed for children.

Refined carbohydrates, such as sugar, give a sudden rush of energy whether we need it or not. These energy rushes from the sugar in carbonated drinks, sweets, and similar junk food products are short-lived, we feel we need more after the rush is over. We become enslaved to extreme highs followed by a slump of energy. This disruption of energy is apparent to parents who have children who don't normally eat simple sugars. When they eat it, they become agitated and demand attention.

There are a number of studies that show there may be a link between alcoholism and sugar consumption. In one such study, Dr. David H. Overstreet at the University of North Carolina commented,

> **Those individuals who reported drinking more alcohol on occasion and having more alcohol-related problems also had problems with controlling how many sweets they ate . . . . They were more likely to report urges to eat sweets and craving for them. They also were more likely to report this craving when they were nervous or depressed, and they believed eating sweets made them feel better.**

Earlier studies comparing the sugar preference among alcoholics showed a similar tendency. When given the choice between five different sugar solutions with varying degrees of sweetness, the 65 percent of the alcoholics preferred the sweetest option as opposed to 16 percent of the non-alcoholics. This is a phenomenon that has been noted by members of Alcoholics Anonymous observed that consuming more sweets diminished the desire to drink. Is it possible that some alcoholics are simply trying to self-medicate?

The natural tendency of soil energy contributes to emotional poise, friendliness, and compassion. If the early emotional life of the individual is influenced by lack of interest, constant criticism, emotional aggression, consistent betrayal of trust, or unreturned affection, these can contribute to an erosion of this energy, affecting both body and mind.

Simple Correctives

The sweet taste is important for health of soil energy, but only when the sweetness does not result in imbalance. The use of fresh fruit, sweet vegetables, and more complex sweeteners can be used to wean the body from simple sugars. The sweetness in vegetables such as pumpkin, yam, carrot, and autumn squash is increased with cooking, especially baking. Cereal grains provide the body with sufficient carbohydrates and, when cooked well, have a mild sweet taste especially when chewed well.

Given the tendency of the character, there is often an attraction to emotional, sentimental, or spiritual approaches to healing. These approaches, if used exclusively, can deflect attention from the more practical methods that could be more helpful in achieving full potential. Exercise, particularly with others, such as yoga, Tai Chi, or Pilates classes as well as social dancing, belly dancing, Sufi dancing, or any activities that encourage movement with friends. The average American consumes an astounding two to three pounds.

Analytical/Introverted (Metal)

Positive Character Attributes

Metal energy characterizes the extreme yang stage in the cycle of transformation. In its constructive aspect, it typifies condensation, accumulation, and the gathering of potential. It is the compression of the resources of soil and the refining of them. Displayed within the individual, this stage of transformation can be seen as a capacity to consolidate experience, to develop self-discipline, and to maintain a generally positive demeanor in their approach to life. This energy is about understanding things and sorting them out.

In the PSI system, they would appear as the "analytical." They are described as quiet, reserved, preferring to engage in one-to-one conversation than with a group. In the PSI system, this character is seen as intellectual, driven by the mind and logic, they need to figure things out—which conforms to the energetic classification. In the PSI, it is also noted that they can be very sensitive to criticism or perceived ridicule.

The Shadow of Metal

What the PSI approach notes is the tendency for the analytic to become gloomy and introverted. This extreme introversion is where the BF system focuses labeling this type "neuroticism." In the energy classification, neuroticism could describe aspects of both metal and water imbalances since both of these character types tend to internalize emotion. Since the direction of metal energy is contractive, this character type can "sink" or "descend" into a depressive state the easiest.

The characteristics displayed with this imbalance are indecisiveness, a feeling of lethargy, and, ultimately, depression. The individual seems unable to cope with even the most minor situations or problems. They often seem frozen or incapacitated, lacking the ability to move beyond adversity. When confronted with difficulty, they are unable to see positive pathways through or around the issue at hand. This confusion of thought leads them increasingly to believe that there is nothing to be done. Unlike the inability to cope expressed in soil, there is less of a tendency to ascribe the fault in the situation to outside influences. The individual is more apt to feel that their inability to act is something wrong with them. They often feel that they are in the way of others and may even feel slightly embarrassed concerning their indecision. They become disinterested in what goes on around them, motivated by a seeming inability to affect events. They may become unresponsive, indifferent, and negative. Once these states settle in, they are not easily disengaged.

When metal energy is stagnated, unnourished, or suppressed, there is a tendency to create a myth of being that is dominated by the thought "I don't matter." They may often seem lost in their own thoughts, engage in activities that don't require interactions with others, sometimes becoming obsessive collectors or hoarders.

Physical Characteristics and Habits

Conforming to the introverted qualities of this imbalance expressive energy is inhibited so that there is a general absence of hand and body movement. There is little or no gesturing; the hands are often stuffed in pockets, hang at the side of the body, or are allowed to lay lifelessly in the lap. There is often weakness in the arms, especially in the ability to lift. The biceps are often flaccid. There is a pulling down and forward in the shoulder areas, producing a kind of slouch that is sometimes accompanied by a jutting forward of the head. The individual may look as if the weight of the world is on their shoulders.

The voice has a tendency to have a slightly monotonous quality or drone. Because of their lack of animation in gesture and speech, others have a tendency to ignore them, which fulfills their expectation of being unimportant and ineffective.

The general complexion tends to be pale and often chalky. This is especially true of the cheeks. In the early stages of imbalance, the cheeks may sometimes appear reddish, with a slight sagging. As these individuals become older, there may be breaking of the capillaries in the area of the cheeks and an extreme pallor in this area.

Meridian Energy

Imbalances in the large intestine and lungs create a corresponding weakness in the muscles of the arms, especially the biceps, around which the lung and large intestine meridians run. Combined with the protective movement of the shoulders moving forward and the correspondent sinking in of the chest, the individual often feels that he/she cannot lift things. Since the large intestine meridian is also affected, there is sometimes clumsiness with the hands, stemming from an inability to coordinate the movements of the thumb and index finger that are controlled by these two meridians.

Physiological Considerations

The energetic qualities of metal animate the functions of the lungs and large intestine. The large intestine is not only a major excretory organ but is also the principal location for the absorption of fluid into the body. Balance of body fluid is of fundamental importance to the functioning of the lungs. If excessive fluid or mucus is allowed to gather in the area of the lungs, then the absorption of oxygen and the release of carbon dioxide are inhibited.

The positive attributes of the metal character are surely an outcome of brain function. While the brain is only 2 percent of the body weight, it will consume between 20 and 25 percent of the oxygen taken in. The brain is very sensitive to oxygen levels, and brain cells begin to die after only four to six minutes if deprived of this nutrient. When oxygen levels are diminished, the result is poor concentration, forgetfulness, mood swings, low vitality, and depressive thoughts.

The word for *spirit* in Hebrew, Greek, Sanskrit, German, French, Chinese, Scandinavian languages, and some Native American languages are synonymous or related to breath. Without proper breath, the spirit cannot animate positive thought or action.

Contributing Factors

The lungs are often obviously influenced greatly by the quality of air we breathe. Breathing has become dangerous in many parts of the world; the fumes of industry and automobiles combined with the diminishing presence of forests and grasslands endanger our health and especially the health of the lungs. In addition to the effects of poor-quality air and smoking, we consume an increased number of foods that produce mucus in the body. Consumption of white flour products, milk, cheese, butter, frozen desserts such as ice cream, and other high-fat foods are damaging to clear respiration.

Any thickening of mucus in the body not only inhibits the exchange of gases in the lungs but also blocks complete respiration through nose and sinus cavities. One of the main culprits involved in this process is dairy food. The promotion of milk products as being essential to health is only challenged by the promotion of meat consumption. The fact that milk creates strong bones is only true for the milk of the particular species. America produces 170 billion pounds of milk each year, and half of it ends up on pizza. In 1970, the average American ate ten pounds of cheese; it is now over 30 pounds. One pound of hard cheese takes ten pounds of milk.

Metal energy can be suppressed in the young by an emotional environment that is too controlled or dominated by others who are constantly in a state of emotional excess or placing forward unreasonable demands for perfection. Too much emotional drama can have adverse effects on the natural desire for stillness and quiet contemplation.

Simple Correctives

Metal energy requires stimulation from good quality yin factors to balance the tendency to contract within. Leafy green vegetables should be used daily as part of the healthy diet described in chapter 12. It is good to concentrate on the more hearty varieties of greens such as kale, collards, parsley, and other greens that do not wilt easily. Mild pungent condiments such as mustard, ginger, or horseradish are helpful especially when eating protein such as beans or fish.

Given the introverted aspect of this imbalance, there is a reluctance to seek help or advice. Contact with new sources of inspiration and good humor can be most beneficial. Aerobic exercises such as swimming, yoga, vigorous walking, or cycling are good to stimulate the lungs as well as yogic breath work. Chanting, singing, or anything that encourages the sustained and expressive use of the voice is helpful.

Creative/Protective (Water)

Positive Character Attributes

The water stage of transformation describes the impetus for movement out of the tightly coiled energy of metal. This is where the yang contraction is released into the yin expansion. There is an impulsiveness that is characteristic of this liberation of energy potential. The positive characteristics of water energy are its adventurous qualities, the release of the potential of the will toward action, and an opening of options. Like water in its physical form, the energy spreads in all directions and is extremely adaptable. It sparks changes in all that it touches and is relentless in its motion. The energy itself manifests in the impulse toward creativity and movement in the individual—the desire to explore.

In the BF classification, the closest match with the water type is called "openness." They observe imagination, creativity, curiosity, and appreciation for the arts, unconventionality, and individualistic behavior as being common in this type. These are all attributes of the water type. The PSI has no match and only list four types—they missed one.

The sense of adventure that is displayed here is accompanied by great willpower and courage. There is an ability to move around obstacles and overcome or "erode" anything that stands in the way.

The Shadow of Water

If water energy is diminished within us, this desire to move out from ourselves is inhibited, and we become tentative in our exploration of the world around us. This disharmony may show itself in anxiety or fear. The individual may feel that the environment is filled with threats and that they are vulnerable and exposed. Their behavior seems overly cautious and self-protective.

Unlike disturbances in metal energy, imbalances here will look outward for an external cause of their problems. There must be some identifying person or object that arouses the feelings of unease. The person does not, however, become introverted; they express their feelings to others and often become physically agitated or emotionally unpredictable.

Physical Characteristics and Habits

Individuals suffering from water energy imbalance often display furtive physical behavior. They may seem anxious, with quick movements and sudden starts. Quite commonly, there is a flitting of the eyes from side to side, a constant surveying, protective in nature, of the space around them. Their body language is also characterized by protective gestures. They tend to be nervous when in enclosed spaces. They prefer to literally have their back to the wall. They like to see everything that is going on so there will be no surprises. They do not like to be taken unaware.

Since water energy is often associated with sexuality, anxiety is often present in dealings with the opposite sex in which case the body language can be very pronounced either being overtly sexual and seeking warmth and protection or avoiding any sexual contact. There is a tendency for the appearance of dark areas of either a blackish or bluish tone on the face and body, specially those areas under the eyes and around the corners of the mouth.

Meridian Energy

Disharmonies in the water stage of transformation create weakness in the meridians of the kidneys and bladder. These imbalances often show themselves most profoundly in a tendency to experience pain, general weakness, and/or tension in the lower back where the bladder meridian crosses over the kidneys.

The bladder and kidney meridians are in close proximity where they move to either side of the Achilles tendon. Individuals with problems in this pair of organs may experience pain or general weakness or stiffness in the ankles or swellings in this area, especially when the kidneys are under stress. Women may experience discomfort in this area during menstruation or pregnancy.

Physiological Considerations

The water stage of transformation is associated with the functioning of kidneys, adrenal glands, the urinary bladder, and sexual organs. The connection here is a combination of three distinct functions, perhaps foremost being the function of the adrenal glands. In terms of the body's internal awareness, if the adrenal glands are not functioning properly, there is a cellular knowledge that the individual cannot respond quickly to any physical threat. There is a diminished capacity of the adrenals to promote the fight, fight, or flight mechanisms of the body. The adrenals also secrete hormones vital to sexual response.

If this is true, it may be that what we are seeing is nothing more than a protective mechanism gone awry. The individuals may then ascribe an external influence to their seemingly illogical apprehension or fear, thereby justifying their feelings.

The final piece in the water imbalance puzzle may well lie in both the energetic and physical functions of sexuality. In Oriental medicine, water energy is often described as ancestral energy—the procreation of our ancestral influences. It is a creative energy and also one involving exploration and adaptability. If this energy becomes stagnated or depleted within the body, then this capacity for external as well as sexual creation is diminished.

Contributing Factors

Water energy is said to carry the capacity for action and willpower, the ability to move through or around difficulty. The kidneys are major contributors to human homeostasis, the optimum body chemistry required for good health. They are responsible for the regulation of water volume in the blood, maintain salt levels, regulate the acid/alkaline balance of blood, and excrete toxic wastes such as urea. There are a number of ways that these functions can be undermined. The first consideration is the quality and amount of water consumed.

The proper hydration of the body is an essential issue in health. All the tissues of the body depend on a proper water balance to transport both nutrients and toxins. As we age, hydration becomes even more important. The issue is best addressed by drinking water, not prepared drinks. The most popular drinks consumed today are diuretics, which means that they encourage urination.

Cola drinks, coffee, alcohol, and any caffeinated drink actually do not address thirst; their main purpose is as a stimulant. The body's natural desire for more water is trumped by drinking fluids that expel rather than maintain fluid. This is doubly confusing for the body since one of the reasons for thirst is to flush away toxic buildup. The imbalance that results is compounded by the fact that an increased number of people work and live in air-conditioned and centrally heated buildings—environments that promote dehydration.

In most macrobiotic books, there is caution against excessive water intake. This is stated since cooked food has a high content of water, and there is a prejudice toward a yang style of eating. For those living an active life and particularly living in cities with a high degree of air pollution, it is important that we have clean water daily.

Combinations of the same factors that inhibit soil and metal can also affect water imbalance. This is particularly true of sugar as commented on above. Sugar depletes minerals in the body and, as a result, affects kidney function. This energy is also poorly affected by the use of cold foods and beverages that shock the system. The use of too much fruit, particularly tropical varieties, are often too expansive and can undermine the integrity of this energy, producing weakness and a lack of sexual and creative energy.

In Chinese medicine, trauma and shock are seen to be especially harmful to water energy and the function of the organs it controls. This effect is particularly true if the events happened in childhood. The sudden loss of a close family member, witnessing a violent event, or suffering from extreme abuse can provide a dramatic shift into fear.

Simple Correctives

The kidneys control the composition of the internal sea of the body fluids. A wide range of trace minerals are needed to nourish the water of the body. In addition to land vegetables, grains and fruits, sea vegetables are exceptionally rich in these trace minerals and are very useful when the energy of the kidneys is low. Sea salt should be used, but in moderation. Beans are also an important addition. While excessive meat protein may cause stress in the kidneys, the proteins found in grains and beans are very nourishing.

People with imbalance in water often feel cold and need not only physical warmth but social warmth as well. Creativity and movement are important for imbalance in this energy. Any creative pastime is useful and is especially good if combined with exercise. Tai Chi, which is dancelike in its movement, is a good example. Joining together with others to do projects such as community volunteer work or groups that share a common interest such as book clubs or amateur theatrics can bring social enrichment and support.

Task Oriented / Controlling (Tree)

Positive Character Attributes

The stage of transformation identified as tree describes energy strongly associated with the spring season. It is the impulse of plants to sprout in the spring and move upward toward the sun. The positive side of tree type is the orderly progression of growth and development. These positive attributes in human character are patience, orderliness, and a general lightheartedness. There is a sense of organization and sense of purpose. It has a strong driving force toward accomplishment, ideas, and social creativity.

Both the PSI and BF systems of character classification identify this particular type with descriptions completely in line with the Five Transformations system. In the BF system, they are referred to as "conscientious" and in the PSI as "dominant" or sometimes as "controllers." They have a high degree of self-discipline, aim for achievement, and are seen by others as being reliable. They have a tendency to be conservative and appreciate exacting and orderly environments. They are natural multitaskers, are confident in their ability to solve problems, and appreciate challenges. They work hard and expect respect for what they do. They like to have a good presentation to public and are often known for being well dressed and image conscious.

The Shadow of Tree

If this energy is blocked within us, these positive qualities turn back on themselves with unpleasant consequences. Disharmony in tree energy can be characterized as overcontrol. When this energy is imbalanced, it leads to rigid, impatient behavior and can be the breeding ground of anger and aggression. The control element is obvious in their own emotional and physical nature as well as their desire to control others. It is easy for them to become frustrated with the perceived incompetence of others. They are often perceived as stuffy, uptight, or workaholics. In the extreme, they can become dominated by irritation, anger, and a cynical attitude.

Physical Characteristics and Habits

Imbalances in tree energy produce the most defensive and aggressive type of body language. This is particularly evident in the muscles of the jaw and neck, with the teeth clenched and the neck muscles rigid. These imbalances are often manifested in hypersensitivity to light and sometimes in eye problems, creating a tendency to squint and producing deep furrows in the brow. There is an inclination for these individuals to hold themselves very erect, and one of the most common gestures is crossing the arms over the chest or lower rib cage. This posture is usually interpreted as a sign of defiance. It is as if they are holding their impatience in.

In communication, individuals with this imbalance have a tendency to speak loudly in order to articulate through their tight jaws and to use sharp, prodding, or cutting gestures with their hands while speaking. There is little fluidity or sense of grace in their body movements. They tend to be look somewhat mechanical when they move. With imbalance in tree energy, the high degree of held tension often is a contributing factor to headaches and stiffness in the joints.

Meridian Energy

One of the reasons for the rigid posture is the tightening of tendons in the body, which is associated in Chinese medicine to the function of this energy. Individuals having these problems tend to sustain injury, swelling, or stiffness in their knees. This can greatly affect their way of moving, creating a type of walk similar to goose-stepping, where the knees have a tendency to lock, and the legs are brought forward with minimal bending of the knee. This type of movement accentuates the overall impression of stiffness and rigidity, and increases the lack of fluidity and grace of the individual in motion.

Physiological Considerations

In Oriental medicine, tree energy is associated with the functions of the liver and gallbladder. There are several possible interpretations of this classification. Of primary consideration is the excessive secretion of bile, which can either be reabsorbed or can back up into the bloodstream. Bile is naturally produced by the liver and is secreted into the digestive system where it is used in the emulsifying of fats for the process of digestion. If bile finds its way into the bloodstream, it can act as a cellular irritant, specifically in its effect on the nervous system, producing a state of persistent irritability. This can be seen in patients suffering from common liver ailments, such as jaundice or the long-term effects of alcohol or drugs where there is often a hypersensitivity to light and irritability of the skin surface. Another symptom cited in Chinese medicine is the connection of tree energy to vision problems.

These symptoms are interesting since they mimic the symptoms of hyperbilirubinemia, a condition in infants caused by bilirubin, one of the substances manufactured in the liver. In some infants, bilirubin is absorbed in brain tissue, resulting in neurological deficits, irritability, abnormal reflexes, light sensitivity, and eye movements.

Contributing Factors

Many of the dietary imbalances in tree energy are caused by an excess of yang foods such as an excess of meat, poultry, hard cheese, or dried salty foods. Over time, the excess of fat and protein creates a hardening of tissue that suppresses the positive qualities of this energy. These problems may be exacerbated by a diet or environment that contains chemical irritants. The fatty tissue of the liver stores toxins when the concentrations become too high. Alcohol and drug use can damage the liver in the same way.

In terms of emotional factors, an emotional environment filled with physical abuse or where there is too much chaos easily reverses the constructive character qualities of tree. Emotional environments where the expression of anger is forbidden can also cause later problems as in the suppression of any reasonable emotional expression.

Simple Correctives

The determined superfocused qualities that typify this imbalance often are seen in their approach to health issues. If they decide to improve their health, they often pick the most stringent dietary extremes and the most challenging exercise programs. This may produce short-term results, but will fail in the long run. The theme for balancing this condition is relaxation for both body and mind. Stretching exercises, relaxation techniques, meditation, and outdoor activities of any type are useful.

In making food choices, it is best to avoid animal foods as much as possible and to eat a wholesome vegetable-based diet. Raw vegetables, lightly cooked, or steamed vegetables help relax the system. Lightly pickled vegetables, sauerkraut, and fermented foods are helpful as well. The use of spicy foods or overly salty foods should be minimized, and fruits should be used regularly.

Extrovert/Erratic (Fire)

The Fire Character

The fire stage of transformation is perhaps the most dramatic of all five. It is often likened to the energy of the sun and represents the height of summer. One analogy commonly used is that tree energy is consumed by fire, radiating warmth and heat and reducing the wood to soil, which begins the cycle anew. The positive attributes of fire are the rhythmic radiation of spirit, a capacity to align the rhythm of actions with the surroundings. The fire type has the capacity to resonate with the rhythm and intent of others while still maintaining a deep sense of self and personal purpose. They are natural communicators and performers and are charismatic.

In the BF system, they are classified under the heading "extraversion." They are seen to have abundant energy, positive emotions, and to seek stimulation and the company of others. They don't mind being the center of attention and are action oriented. In the PSI system, they are referred to as "expressives" and sometimes as "promoters." This type is observed to be able to "light up a room" with their quick wit and often inspirational presence.

The Shadow of Fire

The individual with imbalances in fire energy is often erratic in behavior, flamboyant, and exuberant. They may need attention to gain energy and lose energy when they are by themselves. Their wit can be used as weapons to attack those they feel are a threat. They are talkative and can easily dominate conversations and intimidate others.

There is a tendency to overdramatize situations and to be very dramatic in their expression. This is often extremely appealing to others since they express themselves very cleverly. They can be very persuasive speakers.

In extreme imbalance, they easily lose control of their emotions or be drawn to dangerous, impulsive, and sometimes self-destructive behavior. The need for approval from others may lead them to overcommit to projects or causes. They may often lead double lives being "turned on" when with others and introverted when alone. They do not, however, like others to get too close. It is difficult for them to establish close relationships with many people although they may have passing and superficial relationships with many.

Physical Characteristics and Habits

Imbalances in fire energy can usually be seen externally in a redness of complexion, usually beginning with the nose, which often spreads out into the area of the cheekbones. The nose itself has a tendency to be slightly swollen. It is interesting that circus clowns, known for the extravagant, slapstick humor, often attach red bulbs to their noses for their performances.

In keeping with their extravagance of character, the body language of these individuals is unmistakable, particularly in the use of their hands as a means of communication. There is a tendency to constantly gesticulate when speaking, particularly as the number of people listening grows. The hands are quite often in constant motion, with gestures that move up and away from the body. The gestures are usually well timed with the speech pattern, sometimes producing a hypnotic effect. There is a restless quality in the body language that betrays a lack of internal rhythm and an inability to remain calm.

Meridian Energy

Imbalances in fire energy affect the meridians of the heart and small intestine. These meridians run along the lower part of the arms, with the little finger being their juncture. They control the triceps and can greatly affect the person's grip. The individual may feel a slight weakening or deadening of the grip, and especially when it is cold, a tendency for the little finger to go numb quickly.

Since the natural tendency of fire energy is toward discharge, this contributes to the intricate hand gestures often used by people with this imbalance.

Physiological Considerations

Fire energy is associated with the functioning of the heart, small intestine, and circulatory system. Two characteristics of these systems provide clues to this alignment. One is the function of the circulatory system in maintaining the temperature of the body. This system is responsible for the body's capacity to adapt to changes in temperature in the environment. The second characteristic has to do with the capacity of the heart to adapt its rhythm to changing situations. The heart "keeps the beat" for the rhythm of cellular activity in the body. It is the rhythmic pressure exerted by the heart that presses the blood outward to the periphery where the exchange of nutrients takes place.

A healthy heart should have the capacity to make those adjustments necessary for the increase in blood pressure and its correspondent relaxation. It is precisely these qualities of the rhythm that are not synchronized in the individual with imbalances in fire energy. They are not capable of adapting the rhythm of their own actions to those dictated by their environment. Because they are unable to synchronize their own energy use to a given situation, they unconsciously attempt to dictate the rhythm of events around them to suit their own personal tempo. They feel driven to take control of the situation and to provide the drumbeat for others to follow.

Contributing Factors

The consumption of animal foods and particularly fats has long been associated with heart problems, but the problem goes further. It is the erratic nature of the modern diet and way of life that is most harmful to the energy of fire. The healthy rhythm of the body cannot adapt to the chemical and environmental disarray of modern living. When the balance of yin and yang swings too radically from one extreme to the other, the balance point is seldom experienced. Extremes of diet and activity disrupt the natural rhythm of life, producing extreme stress.

With constant pressure to perform or keep up with multiple responsibilities, a frenzy of activity occurs that is adrenaline fueled. The people with a predication for the fire character will try to master the turmoil and wear themselves out.

Simple Correctives

The key to correcting imbalances in fire is to establish a gentle discipline in life. Following the diet and lifestyle suggestions in the next two chapters could be seen as a perfect approach to bringing fire energy into harmony. The diet should be moderate with a good balance of grains, vegetables, vegetable proteins, fruits, and sea vegetables. Food should be eaten slowly and at regular hours.

Stress reduction exercises, meditation, and gentle exercise are necessary on a daily basis. It is very important that loving relationships with family are nurtured and that arguments and disruptive confrontations are avoided.

The Mutability of Character

I have listed these character types relative to the way they act and appear in daily life. Authenticity of character is where an individual acts out of the positive attributes of a type in their journey through life. They nurture those character traits that serve them and master those that don't. A healthy person may experience both the shadow and the bright side of each quality, but they do not become attached to them. It is when our behavior becomes calcified and thought to be immutable that problems arise. Our attachment to unproductive actions, the habits we develop, is the single most important factor in holding our potential in check. We have the capacity to master our own personal change. When we summon that capacity for transformation into our lives, the latent power of the authentic self rises to meet the challenge.

Chapter Twelve

Creating Balance

Health and Healing

My intention in writing this book was to focus on the implications of creating a healthy life rather than on the details of treating sickness. I hope that I have done that, but do want to comment briefly on the use of macrobiotics as a way of healing specific illnesses. There are many books that cover that topic, and some are mentioned in the reference guide at the end of the book.

Creating health is a reflection of the value that we place on our lives. It is primarily a deeply personal choice. It does not require the assistance of a professional because it simply entails a firm commitment to change. This commitment is not a rejection of assistance, but assistance is only as powerful as our personal resolve allows. There are many problems that we may not have the skill to reverse or treat. There are ways of being that can maximize our health potential, and there are problems that lie beyond our personal ability.

The macrobiotic approach to health involves creating balance in all aspects of our lives. Diet and also some of the practices outlined in the next chapter are self-generated techniques that can be integrated with no supervision. They are things we can do on our own, and they can have profound effect on our well being. How we understand the value of these actions is important.

At the foundation of macrobiotic living is the principle that much of the sickness we experience is a result of the way we eat and live our lives. There is an assumption that healthy actions nourish, strengthen, and enliven us. These actions reduce the incidence of disease, prolong life, and give us increased resources to heal ourselves when sickness arises. It is not a way of cheating death, avoiding age, or completely escaping from sickness. Death, aging, and illness are all part of the human condition. Living a healthy life simply means living to our full potential.

This is based on the understanding that when the body has suffered the abuse of unhealthy living, we are more apt to experience illness and less capable of enjoying our life. When the offending features of that neglect are removed and replaced by healthy influences, the body knows what to do. The body is a self-healing organism, and if given the right resources, it will do what it is designed to do—create as healthy a state of being as possible. It is the body that does the work; we are just making the work feasible.

I have seen thousands of people who have managed to recover their health through the most simple of methods. Many have reversed the symptoms of cancer, heart disease, diabetes, and other potentially fatal illnesses. Even more people have cured themselves of less serious illness such as chronic headaches, digestive problems, sexual impotence, and a wide range of physical and emotional disorders. Their stories are an inspiration and demonstrate how powerful eating well and living well can affect our lives. There are also some that do not succeed. These stories need to be reflected upon as lessons that lead us to an even more effective understanding of health and healing.

The reasons for this variety of response are not a total mystery. The success of healing through natural self-generated means is dependent on several elements: strength of the individual, progression of any illness that may be present, the cause of the illness, diligence of practice, and attitude. Favorable outcomes are generally dependent on the relative strengths or weaknesses in these areas. A major problem lies in the fact that it is difficult to assess these in any consistent way.

I have seen people who have had enormous challenges overcome them and live healthy and vigorous lives. I have also observed those who struggled with seemingly lesser problems and were unable to gain the success they desired. Our approach should be based on common sense, compassion and the willingness to use all the resources available.

The stage of progression of a particular illness is often a great challenge. Many individuals only seek help with macrobiotics or any other natural approach to healing when conventional methods have failed. What should have been the first choice becomes the last resort. I say this not out of a fear or lack of respect for conventional treatment but simply because our cultural approach to healing is so dominated by fear of sickness and a corresponding aggressive approach to symptoms by conventional medicine. In cases of accidental injury, traumatic wounds, serious acute symptoms, or a late diagnosis for a virulent disease, conventional treatment is a sensible choice. It is always possible to establish improved health after an operation or even drug treatment or chemotherapy. Most illnesses do not fall into this category.

Other than living a healthy life before being sick, the first approach to illness should be adjustments to lifestyle. If solutions such as dietary changes, exercise, and stress reduction were promoted with the same energy as medications and surgery, the human and social cost of illness would plummet. We will know when the medical profession is serious about health care as opposed to sickness service when there are cooking schools, yoga studios, and meditation classes in every hospital. These services are inexpensive, effective, and do not require college degrees or medical credentials.

If the problems are more serious, it may be necessary to visit an experienced health counselor to help design dietary and lifestyle recommendations that fit personal needs. This person can also recommend other helpers such as cooking teachers, masseurs, physical therapists, movement or exercise teachers, or stress reduction coaches that can tailor programs for individual needs. The great advantage of these simple techniques is that results can usually be measured in a matter of weeks if not several months. If significant progress is not being made and the symptoms are not dangerous, there is another step before medical treatment.

Acupuncturists, herbalists, and a wide range of health professionals are available to provide specific prescriptive advice and services. These therapies are noninvasive or minimally invasive using natural compounds and generally more sophisticated in their treatment. It is by starting at the most simple and working up that the best results are gained. The first stage allows the person to experience their own ability to manage their life and regulate their health. If progression of the illness has not been curtailed and there are no signs of overall improvement, that is when medical treatment becomes a practical option.

Medical treatment should not be seen as a failure for those following a natural way of life. Using natural approaches to healing teaches us about ourselves and can enhance our life experience, but when it becomes a moral imperative, it often leads to delusional thinking. There is no provable honor in dying or suffering to prove a point. Every problem cannot be solved by diet alone or by any technique, including conventional medicine. It is our choice if we wish to allow our sickness to be a teacher or to pass responsibility for our health to someone else.

Responsibility

It is important that we are able to distinguish between the idea that poor life choices cause many diseases and the idea that a person who is sick has wittingly committed an offense against nature. I have seen this idea raise its head on many occasions, and it is unhelpful and disruptive. We are all ignorant. We are not schooled in the arts of life and not always conditioned to listen to the dissenting opinion, much less the voice within. Our life is open to change at every moment, and at any moment, we may see something previously unseen. In a phrase mystified by former American Secretary of Defense Donald Rumsfeld, "There are things we know and things we don't know and there are things we don't know we don't know." It is the things we don't know we don't know that can create the biggest problems, as Rumsfeld found out. This is especially true when we think we know everything. It is willingness to embrace the opportunity to change and explore the unknown that is important, not what happened in the past.

The dietary and lifestyle suggestions that follow are for making transitions to a more healthy way of life and for health maintenance. The transitional suggestions will increase vitality and produce a greater state of well-being. For most people, the health maintenance suggestions will produce an even higher degree of health as well as improvements for minor ailments. With each refinement in diet, a greater degree of responsibility is accepted. The refined diets used to promote healing for specific conditions are not covered in this book, but a list of books that detail that approach are listed in the reference section. For serious conditions, it is helpful to seek out a professional macrobiotic counselor for advice.

Faith and the Placebo Effect

When we accept responsibility for our actions and begin to change them in the present, the excitement and vitality of health has a chance to develop. This accountability does not place a focus on our past behavior; it is focused on what we will become. We can only be free to mitigate the mistakes of the past when we create a better future through the acts of the present. This is an act of will and an act of faith. Scientific detractors often point to the placebo effect to explain natural healing. This skeptical view deserves a few comments.

The so-called placebo effect is one of the most interesting events in medical science and has been routinely dismissed as an important part of the healing process. The phrase "It's all in the mind" has made it sound like a mental aberration. The logic seems to be if a symptom can be controlled by the mind, it must not be real. Honestly, the placebo is a medical embarrassment.

Researchers at Columbia and Michigan universities demonstrated that volunteers who were told that they were receiving pain medication showed a dramatic release of the naturally occurring pain relieving substances known as opioids in their brains. They were being fed a placebo. These studies were done with sophisticated brain imaging techniques. Other studies have shown that runners who were told that they were drinking oxygenated water performed better even though the water was not treated.

One of the authors of the University of Michigan studies, specialist Jon-Kar Zubieta, MD, PhD, is quoted as saying,

> **This is a phenomenon that has great importance for how new therapies are studied, because many patients respond just as well to placebo as they do to an active treatment. Our results also suggest that placebo response may be part of a larger brain-resiliency mechanism.**

It is estimated that about 30 percent of the population seems to have this ability to respond to placebos. This figure is only reached by assessing direct studies on the placebo effect in drug trials. We all know that the real percentage is higher. Everyone has had the experience of feeling unwell and then being called upon to do something that captures their interest or demands their attention, only to have the pain go away. The human brain is able to suppress pain and speed physical recovery. The placebo effect is all about faith. It is a powerful demonstration of what the internal myth of being can do when motivated. We should wonder about the degree of faith that lies behind drugs as well.

Allen Roses, the vice-president of genetics at GlaxoSmithKline, made a statement that was widely reported in the British press and was received with shock by many people outside the pharmaceutical industry. Many of his associates praised him for publicly stating what is a simple matter of fact among drugmakers.

This is what he said:

> **The vast majority of drugs—more than 90 per cent—only work in 30 or 50 per cent of the people. I wouldn't say that most drugs don't work. I would say that most drugs work in 30 to 50 per cent of people. Drugs out there on the market work, but they don't work in everybody.**

With a 30-50 percent chance of a drug working with possible serious side effects and 30 percent (at minimum) of the population being able to display the placebo effect, with no side effects, we should be studying faith more seriously since it is an important part of healing.

What we have faith in is a personal choice. Our faith has to do with the way we believe life works. Our faith may be placed in a technique, a person, or a higher power, but the most powerful faith is the faith we have in ourselves. This is a faith that can grow when we experience the power of our own ability to effect change in our life. It is the mastery of change that gives us the confidence to trust the miracle of our own creation, the gift of life, and the beauty and power of the natural world we live in. This faith is a demonstration of trust that Creation conspires to create health, awareness, and joy within us when we respect and honor our place in the world.

The Diet Dilemma

I have written in previous chapter about some of the ecological, economic, and health implications of the modern diet. It is time to take a closer look at what would comprise a healthy diet. It is an area that is filled with ambiguity regardless of the force of argument on all sides. The first important distinction we can make is to move beyond good and bad foods. All foods have particular nutritional and energetic qualities. The most important lesson we can learn about food is how these qualities affect our health and the broader implications of their consumption. A food that may be suitable for one person may be harmful to someone else. Some of the foods that we may be attached to have environmental or economic implications we need to respect.

There will be some readers who will be disappointed that there are no lists of "Super Foods," "Miracle Foods," or "Foods That Cure Cancer" in this section. The reason they are not here is that they don't exist. The fact that we are drawn to that kind of promise is that we want nutrition to be like medicine. We crave for the easy answer that doesn't require thinking or personal effort. We want an undemanding approach but are suspicious of simplicity. We crave a miracle but are unwilling to work for its success. The irony is that eating well is simple and can produce positive results; the only precondition is that it requires us to think differently.

One of the less appealing aspects of the contemporary fascination with food and diet is the double-edged sword of food phobias and food and food fixation. While some foods are associated with specific disease, it is usually due to overconsumption of the food rather than the fact that the food is poison. The same is true with the fact that some foods may contain specific micronutrients that are helpful in combating a specific illness. The body is better prepared to redress subtle adjustments in body chemistry than the mind. The balance we crave is best served when we are eating food that is wholesome and not fixating on precision tuning.

The best approach to health is to choose foods that have not been altered with the use of chemicals to the point where they lose their original vitality. To understand the general qualities of foods in terms of their effect on the body, and to consider the broader implications of the use of the foods it is good to have some general principles. In this chapter, there are several criteria that come together in creating food classifications. I have drawn some parallels to a few of the ways these methods of choice conform to nutritional science, but that is not the foundation on which the conclusions rest. The fact that the social, economic, ecological, and health benefits all correspond should not surprise us. When we cooperate with Nature, everyone wins.

Creating Balance

The issue of balance is always present in any discussion of health; the question is, what is being balanced? Obviously, the internal balance of our body and mind is of primary concern. In science, this process of balance is known as homeostasis. Homeostasis is the ability to regulate the internal environment of the body so as to maintain a stable, constant condition. The chemical environment of the body must be kept within certain parameters in order for us to be in good health. This state of balance is of course relative to a number of factors including adaptation to our environment, our activity levels, and other factors that have to do with the challenges of nutrition and the condition of our organs. This is why a sensible amount of experimentation is wise for the person in general good health to locate their zone of personal balance.

Sensitivity is of vital importance in the process of finding balance. The healthy dietary guidelines outlined here are designed to increase sensitivity. After a period of several months, most people will experience a greater ability to distinguish the effects of different foods on their system. As the body becomes used to new foods and a new pattern of eating, it is common to begin to crave the foods you need with an increased sense of awareness. This is the goal—discover by yourself what serves you best. If cravings occur for foods you know are not the best quality, simply choose a replacement, or try the food you crave in small amounts. I suggest that during you initial period of biological education you avoid using dietary supplements of any kind. Taking concentrated nutrients can give you a false picture of what is really going on in your body. If you decide to use any supplemental products after that time make sure they are bio-available and made from plant based organic products. Many vitamin products sold do not digest and simply pass through the system.

An imbalance in our ability to maintain biological integrity can be medically measured by testing the blood or organ function, but this loss of integrity is also perceptible to the individual. We experience these chemical imbalances through the way we feel and by our behavior. Our consciousness can give us the capacity to know when we have moved out of balance if we have some simple criteria to judge by. The usual classification of symptoms of imbalance into yin and yang categories can provide a useful system for understanding personal balance.

The expansive and contractive influences of yin and yang in the body provide the rhythm and harmony of all physical, emotional, and spiritual states. We must breathe in to breathe out, blood has to make its journey to nourish the extremities before returning to the center to discharge toxins and be reconstituted, we need to take in information before processing it as thought, we need inspiration in order to create. This constant flux of energy is the source of our being and shows its presence in every movement of nature.

Imbalances in Yin Energy: Behavioral indications of a yin individual may range from a healthy state to an unbalanced state of being. A healthy yin state could be described as friendly, compassionate, humble, accommodating, or shy. These are pleasant attributes and define a more trusting and tolerant nature. Even though these characteristics reflect a yin quality, they are not disruptive or troubling to the individual or to those around them. It is a nurturing and aesthetic energy more drawn to thought than action. We need both yin and yang to survive.

If the energy of yin is imbalanced, different qualities express themselves. An imbalance of yin is expressed by passivity, lazy, self-pitying, unmotivated, suspicious, fearful, or introverted behavior. The natural receptive qualities of yin become distorted and sink within.

When yin is in a state of imbalance, certain physical symptoms may occur as well. Weight gain in the lower body, swelling of the joints, inflammation, loss of muscle tone, sleepiness, allergies, chronic diarrhea, clear urine, or lack of libido. These are indications of a loosening of the integrity of the body. They are signs that the expansive yin has lost its balance with yang. This is not a medical diagnosis, these are indicators that the body is in a state of imbalance and needs to be pulled back into a more balanced state. They are easily recognized signs that allow us to correct our course.

Imbalances in Yang Energy: The positive qualities of yang are expressed in behavior as being positive, enthusiastic, practical, solution oriented, outgoing, physically active, alert, and self-sufficient. Healthy yang responds with enthusiasm to challenge.

When yang energy is not balanced, it produces tension, rigidity, the desire to dominate or control, lack of humor, material selfishness, and the potential for anger and aggression. The natural desire to create and be an agent of change becomes immersed in greed or contempt for others.

There are often physical symptoms that accompany this imbalance, such as rigidity of muscles and joints, hardening of skin, constipation or hard stools, dark urine, and redness of complexion. The expressive vitality of yang has not been tempered with yin.

Harmonizing Energy: Making balance with yin and yang is simple. It involves stimulating that which is flaccid, warming that which is cold, relaxing that which is tense, and nourishing that which is deficient. Certain foods, emotions, and activities can assist in this process. We all know this. When we are tired, we want to sleep; when we are hot, we want to cool down; when we are stressed, we want to relax. The question is, what do we use to achieve equilibrium, are we conscious of the adjustment, and what are the long-term effects?

If we wish to establish a diet that creates improved health, it is first important to make a transition from the modern diet and create a new foundation to build on. This change in direction is important, and the principles are easy. The healthy diet outlined below conforms to the general description of healthy diets in the Mediterranean, Asian, and North American regions as well as basic macrobiotic principles.

Elements of Healthy Eating

The nutritional elements believed to be essential for a healthy diet are carbohydrates—the main energy source for the body; proteins—for tissue and muscle repair; fats and oils—essential for the use of certain vitamins; minerals—

inorganic elements essential for normal body functions; vitamins—water or fat soluble precursors for many of the body's chemical processes; water—a vehicle for carrying other nutrients and general hydration; and fiber—essential for healthy digestive function. These are the universally accepted requirements for a healthy diet. The only questions that arise have to do with the source, quality, and amount of each factor in producing health.

Creating a personal health plan is about making your own choices. Eventually everyone has to decide what he or she wants to do in order to achieve his or her personal goals. Those goals may simply be to create a diet that is an improvement on what you already do. I hold the belief that if you start to experience improved health and vitality, you will want to stick with what you are doing.

Establishing the Center—Cereal Grains

Any concept of balance must have a pivot point, a fulcrum that supports the outer extremes. In a healthy diet for the planet, cereal grains provide that fulcrum. Whole grains are not only the basis of the human food chain but they also provide the best nutritional complement to other healthy foods. They are rich in carbohydrate and have an excellent protein, vitamin, mineral, and fiber balance. There is no perfect food, but grains come closest.

The invented controversy with carbohydrates has to do with the distinction between refined and unrefined varieties. Whole cereal grains contain all the nutrients of the grain. When grains are broken, some of the nutritional value is lost. Milling grain into flakes, flour, or meal is a process that reduces their nutritional value. Refining the grains by removing all the bran in the outer layer has also removed the essential fiber.

The modern diet has basically confined cereal consumption to white flour. The bread, breakfast cereals, and other baked goods that are familiar to most people have been stripped of nutritional value. In refined flour, an average of 66 percent of the B vitamins, 70 percent of all minerals, 79 percent of the fiber, and 19 percent of the protein has been removed.

The value of complex carbohydrates in the human diet is that they provide a steady supply of energy that is released according to the body's needs rather than flooding the system with sugars not needed at the moment. Part of this slow absorption and release is because they have the range of minerals, proteins, and vitamins necessary for their use. The addition of whole grains as a dietary staple is one of the most important steps to a healthy way of eating.

In the macrobiotic approach to eating grains such as rice, millet, barley, oats, quinoa, wheat, and buckwheat form the foundation of the diet and are recommended for consumption at least twice a day if not at every meal. The use of refined or partially refined grain products such as flour products, pastas, bulgur, couscous, or polished rice are used for variety. Using naturally fermented breads and sourdough varieties are superior to yeasted products, they digest easier and are less mucus forming.

Climate and activity levels should be taken into account when deciding the daily amount of grain to use. For most people, the serving size of grain in the midday and evening meal can be equal or smaller than the amount of vegetables consumed. In hot weather, in warmer climates, or when physical activity is lower, the amount of grain may be slightly less with the addition of partially refined products. Colder weather or increased physical activity may require an increase of grain consumption.

Since grains are not perishable and are there to feed the whole world, eating imported grains is sometimes required to get variety in the diet. The emphasis should still be on consuming those foods that are grown near us or in the same region.

Diversity and Abundance—Vegetables

The use of fresh vegetables daily is a dietary essential. Many macrobiotic dietary suggestions recommend less vegetable intake than grain by portion size. This may be suitable for some, but generally vegetables should be eaten at the two main meals of the day and can be equal or more than the grain portion. The important thing is that there are a variety of vegetables consumed and that they reflect the season of growth as much as possible. It is a good rule of thumb to make sure that you are getting a variety of color in your food. The presence of different phytochemicals such as antioxidants is reflected in plant color. By eating green, white, orange, red, and yellow vegetables over a two- to three-day period, you are assured that you are getting the broadest range of nutrients.

Those vegetables that are hearty, slow to spoil, have less water content and grow in more Northern regions such as broccoli, cauliflower, carrots, onions, parsnips, pumpkin, autumn squash varieties, and brussels sprout are generally classified as more yang. Leafy green vegetables such as kale, collards, daikon radish, bok choy, dandelion greens, turnip greens, leeks, spinach, lettuces, endive, celery, asparagus, radishes, and bean sprouts are classified as more yin.

In summer months or if living in a hot climate, it is important to increase the use of vegetables and to have raw vegetables often. The use of sprouted grains or bean sprouts is a good addition. Leafy vegetables, slightly cooked vegetables or raw vegetables have a cooling effect on the body. Vegetables classified as yin are more beneficial in the heat. In colder climates or in winter, the more hearty yang vegetables and longer cooking methods are good for warming the body.

Organically grown produce, eaten in season are the best choices. Research by the Soil Association in Britain have shown a higher mineral and vitamin content in organically grown food than those grown in chemically treated soil. Soil depletion leads to plant depletion. When adequate local variety is not available, then we must make the best choices with food that has been transported. It is important to support local or regional organic agriculture as much as possible.

The Protein Paradox

In earlier chapters, I have commented at length on the chaos that the meat and dairy industries create. The vast waste of food resources and environmental damage represented in our compulsion to have a meat-based diet is a modern disaster. The move toward a plant-based diet is essential to human and environmental health. This shift in dietary habits can have far-reaching implications for the common good. The most passionate conflicts of opinion among those who eat a natural foods diet are those regarding the use of animal or vegetable sources of protein. It is a discussion that is deeply embedded in both nutritional theory and spiritual morality.

Vegetarian (no meat, only milk products) and vegan diets (no animal products at all) have a long history among various religious groups in the Far East. Hindu and some Buddhist sects have long avoided animal products as an extension of the "thou shalt not kill" principle common in most religions. In modern times, this stricture has been extended to include the mistreatment of animals that takes place in factory farms producing meat, dairy, and eggs.

In the early 1980s, Dr. T. Colin Campbell was one of the researchers presiding over the China Project, the largest epidemiological study of human nutrition that had ever been attempted. The *New York Times* called the study "the Grand Prix of Epidemiology." The study gathered data from 6,500 adults in sixty-five counties in China. The publication of Campbell's book, *The China Study*, in 2005 was a best seller and provided vegans with a powerful nutritional rationale for their practice.

The China Study is a powerful testament to his struggle against the tide of conventional nutrition and the powerful forces of the food industry. His contention that Western nutrition has been ruled by a false doctrine of animal protein superiority is certainly correct. The problem is that the participants in the study were not vegans. His conclusions on recommending a vegan diet were based on the fact that the healthiest individuals ate less animal-source foods. In his words,

> **People who ate the most animal-based foods got the most chronic disease.... People who ate the most plant-based foods were the healthiest and tended to avoid chronic disease.**

It was the amount of animal-based foods that was the deciding factor, not the avoidance of it, that made the difference. This is not to say that an individual cannot be a healthy vegan or that over-consumption of animal products harm health. I have known many longtime vegans who are in excellent health. Many people who follow the macrobiotic principles are vegan. In my health counseling practice, I have also met many vegans and vegetarians, macrobiotic or not, who were in poor health and, in my opinion, could use some animal food as a supplement to their diet. The most vocal opponents of Dr. Campbell neatly illustrate the real health issue at hand.

The Weston A. Price Foundation is an organization devoted to health that bases its philosophy on the studies of Dr. Price in the 1920s and 1930s. Price was a dentist and nutritionist who did fieldwork among pre-industrial populations in Africa, the Pacific Islands, Inuit people, North and South American natives, and Australian aborigines. Among his conclusions were that poor soil, lack of good quality meat, and the introduction of sugar and other refined foods undermined the health of previously healthy people. Dr. Price's observations are very compelling, but do not point to the fact that meat is an essential. What is common to both of the above studies is that if animal-source protein is used, it should be used according to environmental and physical demands. Did the people in Dr. Campbell's study who ate the most meat do less physically demanding jobs? It would make a difference.

We can safely assume that the decision to eat less animal-source food was related to their economic status and not religious principle. Most modern-day diseases are linked to affluence. I know that the tribes studied by Dr. Price were living exposed to the elements and often had scant supplies of vegetable foods available. It could make a difference. The issue of protein needs to be informed by a broader vision than a simple one-nutrient solution.

The macrobiotic view is that animal-source foods are more yang. The energy is more concentrated; they are sourced higher in the food chain. They have already been transformed into animal life and contain the energy of the animal. Because of the concentration of Chi, they are best used with discretion if at all. This does not mean that they are forbidden; it means they demand respect.

Since I know vegans who are healthy, I know that eating that way can work for some. The long-term results of that way of eating are yet to be known since veganism in the West is a recent phenomenon. The most sensible approach if you are eating a diet with meat and dairy on a daily basis, cut it way back. If you are not highly motivated to make a complete change in your diet do it in pieces. Halve your consumption for a month and see how you feel. Eat lower on the food chain, cut out red meat and use more free-range poultry, lower the poultry and use fish. It is a simple and rewarding process.

As dependence on animal-source foods is reduced, add in cooked beans and bean products. Beans have historically been the complement to a grain-and-vegetable diet. Learn to cook them well and begin to use some of the fermented soy-based products such as miso, tempeh, natto, and soy sauce. Use organically made products and try to get them as local as possible.

Bean varieties available in North America and most of Western Europe include garbanzo (sometimes called chickpeas), aduki beans, lentils, black-eyed peas, black beans, great northern beans, kidney beans, navy beans, pinto beans, split peas, and whole dried peas. Soak beans well and cook till soft.

The vegetarian cultures of Asia have developed soy preparation into a fine art. The soybean is very rich in protein but is difficult to digest. Many modern uses of soy are driven by the protein considerations and use soy in products without proper preparation. Using these foods is not a good idea. Miso, shoyu, tamari, tempeh, and tofu are all examples of the natural food processing common in the cultures where they have been experienced for centuries and aware of how they are best used. Tempeh is an excellent protein source and widely available in America and Western Europe. Cooked tofu is a good food to use in moderation. Miso is an excellent concentrated vegetable protein for use in soups and sauces. Long cooking or fermentation makes beans more digestible. The combination of whole grain, a variety of vegetables, beans, and seeds will produce the broadest range of the vegetable-based amino acids essential for protein requirements.

Beans are more yin than grains, but warming in their effect. Increasing bean consumption in the winter months and decreasing them in the summer is a good idea. Some bean products should be used daily in at least one meal except at meals where fish or poultry are used.

Fruits

Fruits are the best source of simple sugars. They are generally cooling and relaxing. They are best used in the season and region where they naturally grow. When living in a temperate climate, it is best for health and the environment to avoid fruits transported from the tropics. The composition of fruits and their sugar content varies widely, the most common northern fruits are apples; they contain 9 grams of sugar per 100 grams while figs contain 19 grams and figs 73 grams per 100 grams. Those fruits with lower sugar content are easier on digestion and contain a more balanced range of the minerals, vitamins, and fiber needed for the buffering and metabolism of the sugars. Fruit is the natural replacement for those eliminating sugar from their diet or for any craving for sweets.

Among the common varieties in North America and Europe are apples, apricots, blackberries, blueberries, cantaloupe, cherries, currants as well as grapes, honeydew melon, peaches, pears, plums, raisins, strawberries, orange, tangerines, and watermelon. More acid fruits such as lemon and grapefruit really belong with the exotics and should be used sparingly.

Fruits are yin and cooling unless eaten in excess. It is a good idea to eat some fresh fruit daily, but not with or right after a meal. Particularly if you have eaten whole grain, allow an hour or so to pass before having fruit or use it as a snack between meals. Fruit relaxes the system. In the winter months, cooked fruit can be used as a dessert or snack. If you are using animal-source food, using fruit daily is an important balance.

Seeds and Nuts and Condiments

The body needs oils to function well. Whole maize, seeds, nuts, and the oil from olives and have been the primary source of that oil for centuries. As used in cooking, oil provides a medium that can quickly sear and seal the outer surface of the vegetable so that it can retain its flavor and qualities as it simmers. Sesame and olive oil are preferred oils since they resist rancidity and provide a good balance of fats. Pumpkin seeds, sesame seeds, and nuts such as almonds, walnuts, and hazelnuts are preferred as roasted condiments or as snacks. Those seeds and nuts that originate in more tropical areas generally have a higher fat content and are more yin.

Macrobiotic condiments such as natural sesame salt, ground seeds, and sea vegetable condiments can be used with any meal. Salt, shoyu, and miso are used to flavor soups and sauces. Pickled plums (umeboshi), natural rice vinegar or umeboshi vinegar are used in making dressings. Common culinary herbs such as basil, bay leaf, cilantro, oregano, mint, and parsley are a nice addition as a change of pace to enhance the flavor of a meal and should be used in moderation. Condiments such as garlic, ginger, wasabi, mustard, or pepper are often used with vegetable or animal protein to stimulate digestion and provide a taste contrast. Pickled vegetables such as homemade vegetable pickles, sauerkraut are an excellent addition to any meal as an aid to digestion.

Sea Vegetables

The use of sea vegetables in Western diets started with their introduction by macrobiotic cooks in America and Europe. Over the years, they have been established as a valuable food group for a healthy diet. These plants have a very wide range of trace minerals at much higher concentrations than land-grown vegetables. They also have the property of bringing out the taste in other foods they are cooked with. Aside from the nori that many people are aware of from eating sushi in Japanese restaurants, there are many other varieties, each with special flavor and characteristics.

Kombu, a flat dried sea vegetable, is an excellent addition to soups or cooked with beans; wakame is used in soups or even in salads; hiziki or arame are excellent for side dishes; and nori can be used as a condiment.

The Exotics

Foods that are classified at the extremes of yin or yang energy are the exotics. They are foods that have a strong effect on the system and need to be used with respect. Sometimes the effect of these foods is not immediately apparent, and sometimes the effect is unpredictable from person to person. They are often foods that inspire addiction because the effect is exciting. As mentioned above, meat and poultry are yang extremes. Most of the exotics are of the yin variety.

Those foods with the most extreme energetic effects are also those that create the greatest environmental and economic harm. Exotic plants are mainly consumed in wealthy countries. They are force grown and usually at the expense of rain forest and small holding farms. Bananas are a good example. They are the fourth largest food product sold on the world market. Growing them to suit the purposes of the West (large size, perfect color, and no spots) requires constant use of pesticides, fungicides, and herbicides that are flushed into local rivers. Since most of the exotics are harsh on the soil, increased use of chemical fertilizers must be used in their growth.

Tropical fruits such as pineapple, mango, oranges, grapefruit, or papaya are questionable for regular use in a temperate climate. Coffee is also a yin exotic. Most tropical fruits have either a high content of sugar or are intensely acidic. Pineapple juice is often used as a tenderizer for meat; it can also remove moles or warts from the body. Hemophiliacs or those with kidney or liver disease are counseled against using pineapple because it can reduce the coagulation of blood. Can we assume that the product that is only dangerous to kidneys if already damaged? If it can tenderize meat, what does it do in the stomach?

Many commonly used exotics are in the nightshade family of plants. These plants have been used for their medicinal properties for centuries. It is an interesting side note that other animals do not eat them. Many of them contain toxins that affect nerve muscle function. Some of these toxic alkaloids can be fatal, and some simply produce irritation. It is well known that they aggravate inflamed joints. Potatoes, tomatoes, sweet and hot peppers, tobacco, jimsonweed, eggplant, mandrake, deadly nightshade, or belladonna are all part of this mysterious family of plants. Cooking has always been suggested for these plants if they are used as foods. Our ancestors knew that cooking reduced the toxins somewhat (by about 50 percent).

Because of their extreme yin qualities, they are sometimes used to relax conditions that have been caused by excessive consumption of animal foods such as meat or dairy. These foods can be looked upon as foods that are used for pleasure or to add variety to the diet but using them in moderation is a good idea.

Do the Dairy Food Experiment

In all the years of working with clients, I have seldom met someone who didn't feel better after three weeks without dairy food take the experiment to two months or more, and you will probably never touch them again. They are extremely mucus forming and contribute to sinus problems in adults and children. Many children with inner ear infections respond quickly to the removal of milk products from their diet.

If you do decide to keep milk products in your diet, simply cut them in half. Go for milk and dairy products that are produced from organic sources, and only use fermented products such as natural yogurt. As mentioned before, dairy farming is environmentally and economically unsound.

Use Natural Sweeteners

Just get everything that has refined sugar out of your diet. Excessive sugar consumption is one of the worst parts of the modern diet. This also means avoiding products that produce the same effect as sugar but are presented as natural options. These include fructose, "natural sugar," beet sugar, brown sugar, honey, and artificial sweeteners.

What about Junk?

Processed foods with chemical additives are not foods that should be used in a healthy diet; avoid them as much as possible. The chemicals used in our foods are experimental. They are used till discovered to be dangerous and sometimes used even when they are known to be dangerous. The FDA studied aspartame, the artificial sweetener, for over fifteen years because animal studies showed tumor production. In 1980, an FDA board of inquiry voted unanimously against its approval. A year later, the commissioner of the FDA, Arthur Hayes Jr., overturned the agency's own scientists and gave it approval for use in dry foods and a year after that approved its use in carbonated drinks. In the year following aspartame, Mr. Hayes departed the FDA and went to work for G. D. Searle who manufactures aspartame.

There are thousands of approved chemicals that are to be found in the weekly diet of people eating the Standard American Diet, no one knows the effect of this toxic cocktail, and no one knows what happens when they go over the threshold from their safe level. We can roll the dice and hope we win, or we can look for a more honest game.

Water

In the attempt to kill harmful bacteria, chlorine is used but is not removed. Chlorine is toxic in concentration. Aside from the chlorine, most municipally-treated water contain other toxic agents, thousands of these chemicals have been found to exist in most American drinking water in "acceptable amounts." Water that is vital, pure, and nourishing is in short supply. The natural cycle of water that includes exposure to the sun, movement over or through stone, and the natural oxidation process of movement in rivers and streams has been altered. The water in our city systems has now been exposed to high levels of pollution, chemically treated and stagnant. Since we are mostly composed of water it is worth paying attention to what we drink and use in cooking.

The movement to bottled water has produced massive fraud, environment waste (plastic bottles), and increased the profits of the soft drink manufacturers who now control most of the bottled water industry. The very least that the educated consumer can do is to buy a simple countertop filtration unit that removes chlorine and other large toxins. There are more complex units available that can reduce or eliminate most of the chemicals from water, and they are worth the investment. If you buy one with a ceramic filter, you will see clearly the amount of sediment that would have been circulating in your system had you drank it from the tap. Use good water for drinking and for cooking, and you will notice a difference. If you feel you need to take water with you to work or play, buy a metal thermos bottle, and don't waste the plastic.

Learning to Cook

Cooking is the basic alchemy of human life. Cooking is the art of combining foods into healthy, well-balanced meals. Cooks know how to improve the digestibility of foods and how to make simple food exceptionally tasty. Macrobiotic cooks have revolutionized the use of natural whole foods in America and Europe. They have discovered how to blend the best elements of food traditions from around the world into a new world cuisine. If you are a novice at using natural foods, you deserve to learn food preparation from one of these men or women.

I have a list of several good cookbooks in the reference section at the end of the book that can give you abundant ideas regarding food combinations and even full meals. Even the best cooks will tell you that the goal is to be able to cook what is at hand with little or no guidance other than the foods that are available, a desire to create healthy meals, and a sense of fun and experimentation. Every man, woman, and child should know how to cook a healthy meal; it is a basic life skill.

Eating

Food is best digested in a calm, friendly environment. Standing up while eating, watching the news, reading the paper, or having an argument is not really respecting the food or the effect it will have. Relaxation aids digestion; it is a good idea to be quiet for a few moments before eating or to offer up thanks for the food. It is the result of many people's labor to arrive on the table as well as the power of creation that is its source. Eating at regular times helps the body regulate the metabolism of the body.

It also helps to chew. If you eat a diet that is rich in complex carbohydrates, the first stage of digestion happens in the mouth. A lifetime of meat eating usually leads to fast eating, carnivores don't usually chew. When a human eats meat, the flavor is gone from the fiber after a few chews. Tell anyone who eats meat to try this out. When you chew grains and other vegetable foods, the flavors last for a long time and often change and become sweeter the longer you chew. Don't become a fanatic; chew well and enjoy your meal.

Remember the point of any modification in your diet is to enjoy life more, not to suffer. We all have a history of food rooted in our culture and family. It is not surprising that we will sometimes crave foods that we ate in the past. Once you have established a healthy way of eating you will find that there are foods that you may enjoy socially with friends or when traveling that lie outside of your new food choices. Simply be aware. Moderate your impulses or have small portions, simple food eaten with distain is no different than extreme food eaten with guilt. It is what you do on a daily basis and in your home that is of the utmost importance. Enjoy!

Chapter Thirteen

Strategies for Well-Being

The Power of Daily Actions

This chapter includes some suggestions and cautionary notes. Some of them are ideas that may be familiar, but familiarity does not need to inspire contempt. You may have already put these ideas into practice; if so, good. I'm sure that there are many more that could be included. The point here is that there are simple acts of health that can be integrated into any life with little training, expense, or difficulty. It is our daily actions that create the pace of our growth. As Robert Louis Stevenson said, "Don't judge each day by the harvest you reap but by the seeds that you plant."

Letting Vision In

Many people are perfectly clear about the vision that enlivens their life; some have an intuitive urge but do not know how to define or express it. If our vision seems hidden or vague, there are simple exercises that we can do that get us moving in the right direction.

Find a quiet place, nature is best, and just sit quietly. Imagine what you would do if there were no restrictions on your actions. Just let those images stay with you for a while. Try to be as detailed as you can—let your imagination go into full flight. Do not edit or judge the images that emerge. If you want, write these things down for later reference. This is a warm-up exercise to stretch your vision muscles.

The second part of the exercise is to be aware of your most precious values in life. What do you stand for? You may not always exhibit these qualities, but they are the ones that are important to you. Write these down and let them settle in.

The third part of the exercise is to imagine your perfect life at its end. This is not morbid; this is your fantasy funeral. Everyone you know and many people you don't know are in attendance; there may even be some famous people there. The funeral is a celebration of your life. It is a review of your achievements and your best qualities. People feel happy to have known you and have been inspired by you. What do they say? How do they sum up what you have represented to them? Since this is all in your imagination, you can do it more than once.

When you have finished this exercise, write down a brief statement regarding your personal vision. Distill all the things that were said about you into a statement of fact about yourself. Make it in the present tense. Allow yourself to be bold. Let that be a starting point. Commit yourself to living by that standard and aligning your actions with that vision. You may find that some of your vision can be divided into different areas of your life: physical, emotional, work, spirit—write it all down. The challenge is not in identifying the vision but acting as if it mattered. You might even want to write down a personal statement of purpose—your visionary job description—and put it in your office or somewhere you see it regularly. Don't be embarrassed.

There is story about the famous psychologist Alfred Adler giving a lengthy interview with a prospective client. After listening to the man's detailed account of his suffering, he asked him what he would do if he were cured. When the man answered him with great enthusiasm, Adler said, "Well, go and do it then." Action is the single missing ingredient in many unhappy lives.

Goals and Action

Creating manageable goals can be an important part in creating health. Your goals should be stepping-stones on your way to realizing your vision. When you review your personal vision statement, you will see that there are things to be done in order to move that vision from a hope to a reality. There may be improvements in physical health and vitality, education, changes in relationships, and any number of personal matters that demand attention. If you look at your life vision as a venture worthy of your time, attention, and investment, creating a plan is common sense.

If you did the simple exercises above regarding what you want your life to be, you will find the seeds for your goals. These goals can be as small or large as you want, but they need to take you toward the realization of your authentic self. They should include actions that you have been putting off till later or have been avoiding because they involved changing old habits or seemed daunting.

If you look at your goals closely, you will notice that they often have smaller actions contained within them. Changing your diet means you have to learn to shop for different foods, you may have to learn to cook, you may have to give away or discard foods you will not need. This means that going to the store, buying a cookbook, signing up for a class, and cleaning out the cupboards are essential steps to doing what you say you want. The next question is when. "Sometime soon" never comes; "when I get around to it" means it's not important. Why not say before Friday? Is this a significant venture or something easily put to the side? You need to know.

Goals without actions are wishes. Action without a plan is often chaos and feeds the monkeys. If we do not make plans and commitments to ourselves, our failures can easily disempower us. If we let our vision fuel our desire, we need to let our plans be the engine that moves us forward.

Positive Self-Talk

Your personal health goals, your work goals, your spiritual goals all have a place here. Choose things that can be done within a particular time frame, say, a month or two, with your best efforts. This is a practice exercise, so don't make your goals impossible. Creating a vision of a healthy life does not mean becoming delusional, but it does mean challenging the limiting messages that we generate within us. The use of positive affirmation is a personal tool that can be of great help in breaking out of the mold of old habits. Make the statements optimistic, focused, and in the present tense. These are self-generated instructions, but they only work well if they are used consistently and with a commitment to accomplishment. Make your affirmations your mantra. Here is an example:

> I am happy that I now only eat food that nourishes me.
> I am excited that I am exercising one hour every day.
> I am delighted that before (fill in specific date) I have finished (fill in project) successfully.
> My daily relaxation and meditation sessions nurture my soul.
> I am grateful for the gift of life.

Make up your own and write your affirmations down and keep them with you, maybe on a card in your pocket where you can touch them as a reminder. Speak them out loud with feeling at least three times a day. You might even want to make a recording of yourself speaking them and play them when you are in the car by yourself—speak along with them and don't give up. If you miss a self-set deadline for a particular goal, reset it—you are the boss. If you don't do it, it never works. Affirmations can help shift attitudes and definitely changes our self-talk. When you have used this for several months, you will find that it is a powerful tool to keep focused on what you really desire.

The direct physical effect of what we think has been extensively studied over the last thirty years. Building on the indications of earlier animal studies, Robert Ader and Nicholas Cohen coined the term *psychoneuroimmunology* (PNI) in 1975. Working with rats, they discovered that the immune function was suppressed when placed under stress. Later studies at Indiana University discovered the connection between the thymus gland and the functioning of the immune system. This has led to the establishment of PNI departments in many major universities.

Aside from the impressive label (with nine syllables), all this tells us something we already knew. Our mind and our emotions affect the way we feel. It would be hard to find someone who has not conjured a headache because of a low bank balance or any piece of bad news. Turning that fact on its head is a major accomplishment. Mind and body are one interactive unit.

Creating a Quiet Mind

Meditation can take many forms, but there are several unifying features. One basic and simple technique is counting breath. Simply sit quietly and count each inhalation and exhalation in your mind. Keep your back straight but be comfortable. Count up to ten breaths and then repeat. Each time the mind wanders and the monkeys take over, simply begin counting again. With daily practice, it is soon possible to keep the mind on the breath and forget the counting; that is when the deep relaxation of mind and body allows us to simply be in the moment. Even ten to fifteen minutes a day can be effective in calming the chatter and ease the mind. Too often, our thoughts are nothing more than an attempt to escape our dissatisfaction with the moment. Our thoughts can become a point of retreat from events that do not fit with our expectations or desires. There is a familiarity with self-talk that provides us with an easy escape from using our intuition.

Whenever possible, experience meditation in the natural environment. When we align our mind with the rhythms of wind in the leaves, the sound of the surf, or any aspect of nature, our minds can experience the deepest spiritual nourishment. Sit by the side of a small stream and pick a stone on the bottom as a point of focus. Do your breathing exercises and place your focus on the stone. When you are completely relaxed, allow your focus to rise up slightly toward the surface and stay there. As distracting thoughts enter your mind, simply release them into the stream and let them float away.

When I was young and lived by the sea, I would go and sit on the rocks or the sand and simply breathe with the rhythms of the waves. When I was upset, I would imagine that the ocean was collecting my teenaged troubles and pulling them away into the deeper waters. It would always leave me with a peaceful mind. The point is that you don't have to follow a particular tradition to start using these tools for health. Use your intention to fulfill your vision and begin to play.

Activity

The four most important factors in the establishment of health are a healthy diet, positive mental attitude, spiritual appreciation, and physical exercise. The body requires physical movement to function at its full potential. Movement enlivens the heart and lungs, stimulates the digestive system, relieves held stress in the body, and stimulates the circulation of Chi energy.

Many of the ancient paths to health included systems of movement that focused attention on Chi energy. Some of these systems have recently regained popularity and combine elements of meditation with movement. Disciplines such as yoga and Tai Chi as well as some forms of Asian martial arts fall into this category. Instruction in these refined forms of movement is widely available, but the important thing is the body is allowed to be flexed and challenged.

The point of productive exercise is not to gain the body of a movie star or athlete. The proliferation of gymnasiums, health clubs, and machines to assist in exercise is often undermining to a healthy attitude toward the body and movement in general. It is possible to overdo it and end up with useless muscle or injury. Unless a man or woman is an athlete, strength training is not essential. The philosophy that it doesn't do any good unless it hurts may work for the professional athlete but is nonsense for most people.

Some of the most beneficial exercises for someone who is sedentary are walking, bike ridding, swimming, or dancing. As fitness levels increase, more demanding activities can be added if desired. The general advice of walking for at least thirty minutes a day would be a great breakthrough for many people. The more exercise is experienced outdoors and in nature, the better.

Like everything else, exercise is about balance. If a person has physical challenges and is weak, simply walking may prove beneficial. If you are tense and stiff, try simple yoga or stretching. If you are weak, try simple strengthening exercises. If you are out of shape and short of breath, try swimming or dancing. Exercise reduces physical stress; improves the circulation of blood, lymph, and Chi; and stimulates good respiration. The more we move, the more we enjoy it.

Sleep

The natural complement for exercise is good sleep. While we sleep, the immune system has time to rebuild, the muscles in the body have the opportunity to release held stress, and the mind is allowed to tap into the deep reservoirs of the subconscious. This is a requirement for good health. Lack of deep restorative sleep is a major contributor to auto accidents, work accidents, and even a major contributor to alcoholism and drug dependence. Deep sleep requires the brain to alternate between deep and shallow levels.

In studies of brain wave activity, it has been demonstrated that delta wave sleep provides the deepest sleep where the body is on automatic pilot and stress patterns disappear. To achieve this state, the alpha and beta waves of wakefulness need to be coaxed to stay quiet. We rise and sink into more shallow and deeper relaxation. The rapid eye movement sleep (REM) is where we dream and have the greatest degree of muscle relaxation. So-called theta bundles, unresolved mental and emotional stress, can disrupt this pattern and prohibit the deeper restorative levels.

Learning to reduce stress through exercise, meditation, and healthy eating is the best solution for deep and healthy sleep. The use of a firm mattress and natural fiber bedding are also helpful to reduce the irritation of excessive heat trapped next to the body and allow the skin to breathe.

Allies and Dream Stealers

As communal creatures, we value our relationships with others and love the camaraderie and support that they can give us. It is a healthy and natural impulse. We want our friends to be trustworthy, honest, and supportive of our life vision. Ideally our friends and family are filled with goodwill toward us and have some degree of alignment or respect for the way we wish to live our lives. They also want the same from us in return.

The closer that mutual bond of affection becomes, the more it contains an element of protectiveness both toward the friend and toward the relationship. We don't want our friends to be hurt. There is an interesting adjustment to be made when one individual makes significant changes in their life. Those changes may be perceived as dangerous to the bond between them. This is not always a conscious attitude; it may simply be a sense of unease. It is not unusual for one party to feel that their friend is on a dangerous path or that they are in danger of being left behind.

This may seem an unimportant issue, but for many, it is not. In *Hamlet*, Polonius instructs his son before he leaves for his travels, "This above all: to thine own self be true, and it must follow, as the night the day, Thou cans't not be false to any man." Well said, Shakespeare. This is good advice for anyone as long as we are aware that the truth as we see it has a nasty habit of making waves. It is only through respecting other opinions while not being bound by them that disruptions can be minimized. A friendship or any relationship without honesty is sailing in dangerous waters.

When our actions or opinions run contrary to our social group, there are many friends that will simply become observers to see how the changes turn out. The relationship is unchanged, and there is simply a new element. Interesting discussion, debate, or curiosity are all good responses. This is how it should be. Problems only arise when the changes are seen as challenges or presented as confrontation.

I have seen many people who are attempting to integrate a new way of eating into their lives who manage to insult their friends and families by insisting that they have discovered the Holy Grail. Patronizing behavior and defensive argument are not signs of a healthy life. The vegetarian or "macrobiotic" person who feels compelled to criticize others for their diet should take a deep breath and reflect on why they have the need for others to bend to their will. When we are "being the change we want to see," we must allow others to make their own choices. This does not mean hiding or concealing what we do. Our own commitment needs to stand on its own.

There are some people who have absolutely no interest in the things that interest me. There are those that want to argue. There are some that may be curious and ask questions; and there are some that are ready to change and are looking for guidance, information, or support. There are also those who are walking the same path and have their own insights and experiences to share.

We will never open the closed mind; it is a waste of time and energy to attempt it. Everyone has their own vision of life and their own capacity to change if they wish. Not everyone moves at the same pace or in the same direction, that's yin and yang. I have friends who live very different lives than I do and still have qualities that I respect and can learn from. If they are interested in any of my eccentric ways, they will ask. There are many seekers in the world, and if we hold to our own truth, they will present themselves to us. That's the way the world works. Coincidental meetings, fortuitous events, and intuitive discoveries are a side benefit of a healthy life. Our alignment with nature will often take us exactly where we need to go.

I found myself in Southern France on New Year's Eve 1970. The city was celebrating, and I was on my own. I had been staying in hostels and pensions, cooking for myself. Given the celebrations of the evening, I decided to give myself a treat and find a restaurant where I could get something special. As I was walking down the street, I noticed a neon sign advertising Vietnamese food and thought I might find some rice and vegetable dishes. Inside the empty restaurant was a smiling woman who showed me to a table and gave me a menu.

Using my French dictionary, I was trying to figure out what to eat when I noticed a small sentence at the bottom of the menu with the word *macrobiotique*. I called the woman over and pointed to the word and asked what it meant. She became instantly excited and called into the kitchen and out came the cook. With his little English, he told me that his family had met George Ohsawa in Vietnam many years ago, and he had helped their father with his health. Since they were restaurant owners, Ohsawa had made the father promise that they would always put a mention of his diet on the menu in case a hungry traveler came their way. They had not had that hungry traveler for decades. I enjoyed course after course of wonderful food served with great affection and good humor. The wine came out, the radio was turned on, and we all ate together. There were no other guests the whole evening. Just a coincidence.

Allies come in all shapes and sizes. They come when we least expect them, often disguised as innocent bystanders, sometimes as new acquaintances. Allies can help us on our path; they may shine light into the dark corners or challenge us to be true to our own vision. They may teach us a new skill, enliven our thinking, or simply support us in times of trouble. It is our own energy and engagement that will draw them to us.

Allies are the exact opposite of dream stealers. Dream stealers do not want us to change because they fear it. They will ridicule that which they don't understand or attack to protect values that seem a danger to their thoughts. They are not open to discussion but thrive on argument. The energy of their opposition is usually driven by fear and insecurity.

I have seen dream stealers undermining attempts by family members who are improving the quality of their life even in the face of obvious success. If friendship does not include mutual esteem, it is not friendship. This does not mean continual agreement or mindless support; it means respect. A friend may disagree with your plans but respects your choice once the objections are raised. The dream stealers do not respect; they demand conformity on their own terms as a condition of friendship. They are not agents of change; they are guardians of orthodoxy.

Dream stealing lives not only in individuals but also in institutions. The popular press is filled with dream stealing. The cynical assessments given to global warming in the past decades, the suspicion of organic agriculture, and many of self-serving cautions regarding the dangers of social and individual change are largely based on panic. The movement from "having" to "being," respecting the environment, and even establishing health are revolutionary and essential. Supporting a larger vision of human potential requires an unwavering will and an open heart.

Unplugging

Being available day and night for work-related e-mail or cell phone access seems to be a badge of importance. It conveys a sense of personal value and indispensability. I often see people doing business on vacation or while they are at the playground with their children. I have come across men using their cell phones in the high mountains when they could get a signal and even in the middle of a river while fishing. The point is not about the cell phone or the laptop. The point is that our lives become increasingly dominated by the technologies that were meant to create freedom and instead produce a kind of slavery. It is a slavery that pulls us out of the surrounding environment and into the techno-space. It is a slavery that pulls us away from being in the present, away from the flux and flow of life around us, and into a virtual world.

The web of energy that most modern people are linked to is not nature but media. Instead of the flow of Chi through the elements, we are linked most intimately to the electronic pulse of television, radio, cell phones, iPods, and the Internet. The average American spends more time using media during their waking hours than any other activity. A study at Ball State University discovered that the average person spends about nine hours a day using some type of media. Even using my meager skills at math, that means that eight hours of sleep and nine hours on media equals seventeen hours—only seven hours left for everything else.

Initially I thought they must be wrong and then remembered my last visit to America. There were TV sets in many restaurants, sometimes several channels with the sound off. There were TV sets that could be watched as you checked out at the supermarket, there were TV sets in elevators, and every store had music playing. I know that in some homes the television set is never off if there are people in the house. I had to review my skepticism. I can hear some ask, "So what?"

If the source of our existence pours through the organic life-forms and natural elements of the planet, it is important for us to be in touch with those forms. The stillness of the mind, the awareness of our body and our thoughts, and the presence of others is easily drowned out by the static of information passing through the group monkey mind. It is not about rejecting technology but about creating space for humanness. The more we are surrounded by media, the more we are ruled by mediocrity. Discernment is essential. Learning to unplug is a healthy thing to do.

Emotion

While I have placed focus on the effects of general health, diet, and other factors in creating health, I have not discussed the role of emotion except in character type. There is no question that emotional events influence us greatly and can color our vision of life. For many people, the emotional landscape is where all the important events take place. Each person has to decide what path they take to establish health and to accelerate healing. This book is no more about addressing serious mental illness than it is a book on curing cancer. Serious problems require professional help. The issue of emotion in healing is a popular one and needs some attention.

Emotional traumas caused by harmful actions to our person or by witnessing an event have an immediate and long-term effect on the body and the mind. This is also true regarding positive experiences. Our brain stores these experiences and remembers them. They can be called up by exposure to a person associated with the event, a smell, weather, a tone of voice, or any number of triggers.

If there is a powerful disruption in Chi flow caused by emotional events, it can be reflected in the body as a bioenergetic blockage associated with organ function. Realigning these energetic abnormalities can be facilitated in many cases through therapeutic massage, bodywork, or acupuncture. Other therapies or exercises done in one-on-one or group settings can be helpful in increasing awareness of how we hold these memories and be helpful in allowing us to defuse the power that they have on us. There is a fine line between acknowledging past problems and being ruled by them.

Most people have witnessed bad things happen or experienced them firsthand. The past is unchangeable. The idea that we can dismantle the past is a fallacy, and revisiting it is not always a wise course of action. Consistently revisiting the past and picking it apart often empowers it and strengthens its ability to control the present. It is in the present that we exert the most control over the future.

Establishing healthy habits of mind, body, and spirit will challenge the energetic, emotional, and physical patterns of the past and are a positive way of incorporating them into our being so they lose their power. The self-centered idea that we can wipe the slate clean of past misfortune only profits those who promise to accomplish that miracle. Emotional health is not rejecting the past; it is accepting it as exactly what it is—the past. Past emotional wounds cannot be healed, only disempowered.

Education and Creativity

Education is a process that should never end. The word *education* has been defined as deriving from the Latin *educare*, "to rear or to bring up" or to "pull out" or "lead forth." The important distinction here is that education is not about putting in; it is about bringing out. Education calls forth our imagination, our curiosity, and our native potential to grow. We are either growing or dying—life has no convenient grey zone. There is no middle ground. Education means we are experimenting and finding out new things about the world and our place in it. This can only happen from the inside out. Experience is the greatest teacher and is dependent on having a rich diversity of exposure to ideas and events.

Learning to navigate the shifting tides of change in our daily life is the bedrock of wisdom. When we are aware of the changes that take place as we create improved health, we are learning the laws of nature in a powerful and intimate way. The lessons we learn will help us in every aspect of our lives. The energy that we obtain from this process is enlivened when we express it.

Health requires expression. This is where creativity and action enter the picture. If we have an exciting vision for our lives and have set goals for its realization, we need to follow our vision with enthusiasm. Find out what you love and do it. The American mythology professor, writer, and lecturer Joseph

Campbell counseled his students to "follow your bliss." This phrase simply condenses the most profound aspirations of healthy living.

Our culture has become lazy where personal education is concerned. I have often encountered clients who are sick, realize that there are simple things that could improve their condition, and refuse to do them because they find the challenge of learning something new stressful. If we balance heart disease with learning to cook or a lifetime on drugs against exercising every day, which option wins? You might be surprised. Learning new life skills can be an adventure or a struggle; the only defining factor is the volume of monkey talk and the strength of our commitment.

If we do not pursue our goals and visions now, when will we do it? It is only monkeys that hold us back. The proving ground for the improvements we want to see in the world around us must begin with us. Human life has become the single problem that faces the planet, our children, and ourselves. Only when we anchor our transformation in our own lives do we become fully empowered to effect the changes we wish to see in the world.

(Author's note: I want to say that for the record, I find monkeys a fascinating tribe of creatures. They are witty, entertaining, affectionate, and resourceful. My statements about the monkeys in human heads are only imaginary. Any similarity to real monkeys either living or dead is purely coincidental.)

Home Environment

Where we live is our sanctuary; it is where eat, think, sleep, meditate, and create our dreams. It may be an apartment or a house, it may be humble or grand, but it should always support a healthy life. The art of feng shui, the Chinese study of placement, has become popular in recent years and reflects centuries of study on the way that the energy of a living or working space can affect the occupants. I have been in homes that looked like an Oriental temple or a Zen monastery after following the advice of a feng shui consultant; this misses the point unless that design makes you comfortable. Comfort is important as well as pleasure to the eye, but these are often cultural values. Our home will reflect our character but can also help us to establish a clearer mind.

I once visited a client who I knew had experienced a troubled childhood and a lifelong struggle with her parents. I was surprised that her home was filled with furniture and objects that she had inherited from their estate. This was the debris of an unhappy period of her life and had become a fortress that confined her in past misery. It was a physical representation of her inability to let go and move on. I proposed that she let it all go. Her reluctance to sell it all and redo her apartment was a major healing crisis for her.

She cried and became very agitated and even angry that I would suggest it. When she eventually decided to "clean house" and to create a space that reflected who she was becoming rather than who she had been, the change in her was amazing. She brightened her mood, became clearer in her mind, and even felt that her physical condition improved.

The first principle of a healthy home is to reduce that which is unhealthy. Cupboards that have poor-quality foods from past habits need cleaning out. A clean kitchen and cooking utensils help to create better food preparation, clean windows let in the light, and a clean house enhances relaxation and sense of self-respect.

Clutter is one of the things that can burden us down and even anchor us in the past. I am always amazed at the amount of unneeded paper and stuff that I manage to collect. If things are not being used, recycle them or give them away. By reusing, recycling, and reducing what we use, we become more respectful of what we have. It is not essential to live the life of a monk or live in voluntary poverty, but simple is good. Discernment is the issue.

According to many environmental studies, the air inside houses is often more polluted than the air outside. A frequent airing out of living spaces is a good idea as well as getting rid of toxic materials stored under the sink or in storage cupboards. Many chemical cleaning solvents leak toxic fumes into the air in houses. Plants help to keep the air fresh (if you water them and treat them well), and when you are able, air filtration units can be a helpful investment. For many years, I have used a simple filter and am always amazed at the amount of debris that collects in them. Even very clean homes have dust, microorganisms, and particles that are free floating and inhaled. They are especially effective in the bedroom and for those who have respiratory problems. There are many good products on the market, and some even kill the microorganisms in the air.

The pursuit of simplicity and health can be reflected in all our choices. The transportation we use, the foods we buy, our use of electricity, our choice of clothing can all be informed by our ideals without depriving ourselves of a comfortable and pleasant life. The opinions to the contrary are only feeble excuses to avoid personal commitment.

Bonding with Nature

At the very beginning of this book, I talked about my personal sadness at the disappearance of the rivers and forests of my youth. This process of pillaging the environment that is the source of our lives should make us all pause and reflect on our own unwitting contribution to this horrible error in human judgment. Our neglect of the environment is an act of self-loathing, a matricide of epic scale. Stopping and reversing this illness of body, mind, and spirit requires a new consciousness, self-discipline, and increased honoring of the natural world.

Establishing health while living in modern society is a revolutionary act that can assist in the process of healthy social development. It helps to anchor our ideals in daily action and increases our capacity to feel the connection with the world around us. This connection is the spiritual link between the larger flow of energy that enlivens the world we live in and ourselves. This is not an act of self-sacrifice—it is an act of expanding the vision of who we are.

The tribal teachings of the aboriginal peoples of Australia tell them that their songs bring the world to life. As they walk the pathways that were walked by their ancestors, they sing ancient tribal songs. These songs describe the landscape they are moving through. Every spring, tree and rock formation is part of the song. These songs were ancient methods of navigation in the outback. They are singing the land into their consciousness; the world is alive within them. Their legends tell them that if they stop the songs, the world ceases to exist.

Human beings have the power to place value in the world. The aboriginal teaching empowers the individual not only to appreciate the worlds outside and within but also to make conscious the bond between the two. It is a way of being which promotes constant reflection on the relationship we have with creation and our place in it. The songs, the poems, the stories of the past speak to the connectedness of all things. I want to leave you with a poem, by the American poet and naturalist Gary Snyder, that I have often used in workshops and seminars I have given. I hope that the beauty of it reminds and rekindles the desire to breathe new life into Mother Earth and the awesome power of creation that lies at the source of all life. It is time to sing the world alive again.

Prayer for the Great Family

Gratitude to mother earth, sailing through night and day—and to her soil:
rich, rare and sweet
In our minds so be it.

Gratitude to plants, the sun facing light changing leaf and fine root hairs;
standing still through wind and rain;
their dance is in the flowing spiral grains.
In our minds so be it.

Gratitude to air, bearing the soaring Swift and the silent Owl at dawn.
Breath of our song clear spirit breeze.
In our minds so be it.

Gratitude to Wild Beings, our brothers, teaching secrets, freedoms, and ways;
who share with us their milk;
self-complete, brave and aware.
In our minds so be it.

Gratitude to Water: clouds, lakes, rivers, glaciers, holding or releasing—
streaming through all our bodies salty seas.
In our minds so be it.

Gratitude to the sun: blinding pulsing light through trunks of trees, through
mists, warming caves where bears and snakes sleep—he who wakes us.
In our minds so be it.

Gratitude to the Great Sky
Who holds billions of stars—and goes yet beyond that—beyond all powers,
and thoughts and yet is within us—Grandfather space and the Mind is
his wife.
So be it.

Gary Snyder (after a Mohawk prayer)

Useful Books Inspired by Macrobiotics

The Macrobiotic Path to Total Health by Michio Kushi and Alex Jack
Publisher: Ballantine Books

The Do-in Way: Gentle Exercises to Liberate the Body, mind, And Spirit by Michio Kushi
Publisher: Square One Publishers (August 6, 2006)

Your Face Never Lies (Avery Health Guides) by Michio Kushi
Publisher: Avery (May 1, 1983)

Modern Day Macrobiotics by Simon Brown
Publisher: North Atlantic

The Great Life Diet by Denny Waxman
Publisher: Pegasus Books

Nature's Cancer Fighting Foods by Verne Varona
Publisher: Reward Books

The Energetics of Food by Steve Gagne
Publisher: Spiral Sciences

Essential Ohsawa by George Ohsawa
Publisher: George Ohsawa Memorial Foundation

Cooking the Whole Foods Way by Christina Pirello
Publisher: Penguin Group

Glow by Cristina Pirello
Publisher: Penguin Group

American Macrobiotic Cuisine by Meredith McCarty
Publisher: Avery Publishing Group

Fresh From a Vegetarian Kitchen
Publisher: St Martins Griffin

Sweet and Natural by Meredith McCarty
Publisher: St Martins Griffin

Marlene Macmillan's No Nonsense Guide to Healthy Living by Marlene Macmillan
Publisher: Grosvenor House Publishing

Karma Cookbook by Dragna Brown and Boy George
Publisher: Carroll & Brown

INDEX

A

Ader, Robert 157
affirmations 157
airing of living spaces 166
alcohol 69, 89, 92, 102, 110, 123, 130, 132-3
anxiety 27, 34-5, 58, 96, 121, 128
Ardrey, Robert 99
Armstrong, Karen 21
authentic self 26, 28-9, 42, 44, 51-4, 59, 60, 63-6, 72, 74, 76, 115, 136, 156

B

balance 57-8, 66-7, 75, 81, 97, 101-2, 104-5, 107, 114-5, 127, 136, 142-5, 150, 159
beans (*See also* vegetables *under* pyramid *in* food) 90, 92, 99, 102, 104-6, 127, 130, 146, 148-50
Besser, Richard 86
Bohr, Niels 26
boredom 70-1
Britain on the Couch 32

C

Campbell, T. Colin 147
Castaneda, Carlos 74
Chi 43, 62, 65-7, 107, 112, 115, 119, 148, 159, 163
China-Oxford-Cornell Diet and Health Project 91
China Study, The 147
Chinese medicine 13, 55, 62, 109, 112, 120, 130, 132

Cohen, Nicholas 157
Confucius 20-1
consumerism 32, 34, 37
consumption 13, 31-2, 35, 47, 52, 54, 83, 90-1, 96-7, 99, 104, 106, 122, 142, 145, 148
convenience foods 88, 97-8
cooking 77, 96-8, 102, 123, 148, 150-1, 153, 161, 169
Csikszentmihalyi, Mihaly 37

D

Dawkins, Richard 63
de Mille, Agnes 68
death 19, 28, 31, 37, 43, 48, 50-1, 85-6, 103, 137
Department of Health and Human Services 85
depression 32-3, 58, 96, 118, 120, 124
diamon 73
diet 12-3, 42, 50, 52, 54, 57, 64, 77, 81-3, 85, 87-8, 91-3, 95-104, 106-11, 122, 127, 133, 135-7, 139-42, 144-52, 154, 156, 158, 161, 163
digestion 95, 98, 106, 111, 132, 149-50, 154

E

Eckhart, Meister 26
emotions 12, 20, 38, 44-8, 57-8, 60, 65, 75, 93, 109, 117, 120, 127, 133-4, 144, 158, 163
enchantments 17-8, 29, 32, 35, 40-1, 46, 75-6, 84, 92, 98, 117

energy 22-3, 38-9, 43, 46-7, 51, 54-6, 60, 62, 64-8, 81, 93, 96, 98, 101, 103-4, 111-5, 119-20, 122-4, 127, 129-36, 138, 143-5, 148, 161-5, 167
  creative 129-30
  cycle of 116, 120
  expressive 125
  molecular 23
  spiritual 43, 76
  stored 122
Environmental Protection Agency 90
epidemiology 83, 147
exercise 47, 55-7, 69, 84-5, 90, 124, 130, 138, 155-6, 159-60, 164

F

faith 18-9, 29, 60, 71, 84, 96, 140-1
Falwell, Jerry 19
five phases. *See* five transformations
five transformations 114-5
  fire 114-5, 133-6
  metal 114-5, 124-7
  soil 114, 120-1, 123-4
  tree 114-5, 131-3
  water 114-5, 127-30
food 5, 9, 13, 17, 23, 25, 29, 31, 37, 39, 40, 43, 52, 54, 56, 60, 66-8, 73, 76-7, 81-5, 87-93, 95-112, 122-3, 126, 130, 133, 136, 141-54, 156-7, 161, 166, 169
  industry 13, 83-4, 87, 89, 92, 97-8, 147
  pyramid 92, 102
    bread 37, 77, 145
    dairy 89, 90, 101-2, 108, 147-8, 151
    fruits 89, 91, 99, 101-6, 130, 133, 136, 149-50
    meat 89, 92, 98-102, 105-6, 133, 147-8, 151, 154
    poultry 133, 148-9, 151
    sugar 89, 92, 95, 97, 102, 105-6, 108, 122-3, 130, 145, 148-9, 151-2
    vegetables 77, 89-92, 99, 101-6, 108, 123, 130, 133, 136, 146, 149-50
Fromm, Erich 31, 33-4, 36

G

Gaia 23-4, 26, 36, 43, 45, 64, 81, 119
goals 31, 38, 42, 47, 52, 67, 71-6, 143, 145, 153, 156-7, 165
"Good and Bad Reasons for Believing" 63
Govinda, Lama Anagarika 66
Great Transformation, The 21

H

habits 12-3, 48, 52, 59, 69, 70, 74-6, 88, 100, 110, 113, 121, 125, 128, 131, 134, 136, 156-7
happiness 27, 31-5, 37-8, 40, 42, 69, 83
To Have or To Be? 31
health 5, 12-3, 15, 18-20, 23, 29-31, 36, 41-2, 50-8, 63, 67-72, 76, 81-6, 88, 91, 93, 95-9, 101-5, 109-11, 113-6, 118-9, 121, 123, 126, 129, 133, 137-45, 148-9, 155-6, 158-9, 161-4, 166, 169
  emotional 44, 164
  environmental 12, 34, 147
  qualities of 51-4
  spiritual 42, 64, 66
Heraclitus 61
Hillman, James 73

I

imbalances 51, 55-9, 67, 82, 87, 93, 96, 101-2, 119-20, 122-5, 127-8, 130-3, 135, 143-4
  five transformations 128, 144
  stages of 55-9

J

James, Oliver 32
Journal of the American Medical Association 86

K

Kassar, Tim 34
Kushi, Michio 13, 104, 169

L

Lappe, Frances Moore 89
Lovelock, James 23, 36

M

macrobiotics 13, 54, 57, 67, 72, 77-8, 95, 103-5, 107-9, 137-8, 146, 148
Macrobiotics and Human Behavior 109
Maslow, Abraham 42
milk 82, 89, 101, 104-5, 126-7, 152, 168. See also dairy *under* pyramid *in* food
Morris, Desmond 99
myth of being 28, 117, 125, 141

N

New Scientist 32
nutrients 25, 82-4, 87, 92, 96-7, 107, 111, 126, 129, 135, 145-6
  carbohydrates 82, 102, 124, 144-5
  fats 82, 84, 92, 97-8, 101-2, 132-3, 135, 144, 150
  fiber 92, 102, 145, 149, 154
  minerals 24-5, 82, 102, 104, 130, 145-6, 149-50
  protein 60, 82, 92, 101-2, 104, 130, 133, 144-5, 147-9
  vitamins 50, 82-3, 102, 144-5, 149
nutrition 37, 54-6, 60, 82-5, 87, 91, 103-5, 122, 142-3, 145, 147

O

Ohsawa, George 13, 41-2, 51, 57, 59, 66, 105, 108, 161
oils 36, 89, 105, 144, 150
Orwell, George 39
Overstreet, David H. 123

P

personality typing
  Big Five system 118-20, 124, 127, 131
  Myers-Briggs Type Indicator 118
  personal style indicator 118, 120, 124, 128, 131, 134
"Prayer for the Great Family" 167
Price, Weston A. 148
Psychopathology 96

R

Roses, Allen 141

S

Schumacher, E. F. 63
sleep 52-3, 56, 159-60
soybean-based products 106, 149. See also vegetables *under* pyramid *in* food
Stenger, Victor J. 111
stress 11, 13, 37, 52, 54-7, 67, 74, 104, 107, 116, 122, 129, 157, 159-60

V

vision 13, 18, 20, 28, 30, 34, 36, 40-2, 46, 48, 51, 53, 71-7, 96, 100, 102, 109, 112-3, 148, 155-8, 161-5, 167

W

water 11, 13, 23-5, 30, 32, 43, 53, 55, 60, 62-4, 66, 70, 81, 90, 93, 96-7, 106, 111-2, 114-6, 127-30, 140, 145, 153, 158, 166, 168
Wilson, E. O. 19

Y

yin and yang 43, 60-1, 64-5, 67, 101-2, 105-7, 114-5, 120, 133, 136, 143-4, 146, 148-51, 161